ADVANCE PRAISE FOR *MORE THA*

As Minister of Health, I was pleased to take part in the Ghana model training program, which we adapted and implemented successfully in Ethiopia. As WHO Director-General, knowing what countries need, I recommend this book for individual learners and academic institutional leaders who want to develop and participate in collaborative, mutually beneficial, and sustainable global health training and education.

—Doctor Tedros Ghebreyesus, Director General, World Health Organization

Doctor Johnson, who found a moment of compassion, clarity and action during an unexpected trip to Ghana, and subsequently went on to lead the development of life-changing, life-saving collaborations in women's health care between U-M and several universities in Ghana, has produced a remarkable work, a memoir, a blueprint, and an exhortation to action. It's an important read for anyone interested in practical solutions for reducing global health inequities, and for all those who strive to live lives of compassion, innovation and impact.

—Santa J. Ono PhD, President, University of Michigan

More Than "First, Do No Harm": Academic Global Health is a must-read book for practitioners, researchers, academics, development workers, policymakers, and philanthropists. Professor Timothy Johnson impressively chronicles the enduring success of The Ghana Postgraduate Training Program in Obstetrics and Gynaecology in improving women's health in Ghana and in becoming a role model for medical schools throughout the African continent and elsewhere. With lively description, Johnson illustrates the importance of sustained vision, leadership, and teamwork—as well as international, national, and local support—in building effective academic health programs with practical and lasting benefits.

—Patricia L. Rosenfield, PhD, author: *A World of Giving: Carnegie Corporation of New York-A Century of Philanthropy*, and former chair, Carnegie Corporation's Strengthening Human Resources in Developing Countries Program

Chronicling his decades long commitment to global health, with a focus on Ghana, Johnson shares insights and lessons learned that have broad applicability to all North–South relationships. Richly augmented with interviews with multiple faculty, trainees and leaders from both North and South participating institutions, *More Than "First, Do No Harm": Academic Global Health* should be on the reading list for all currently involved in or considering North–South University relationships or indeed work in any low resourced setting.

— James O. Woolliscroft, MD, MACP, FRCP Professor Emeritus of Internal Medicine and Learning Health Sciences Dean Emeritus, University of Michigan Medical School

I am told that in Ghana, it's important to know who someone's father is. It provides context, reassurance, and a degree of familiarity that smooths interactions from then onward. A Ghanaian colleague once told me, "For all of you from the University of Michigan, when you are in Ghana, Tim Johnson is your father." I think that speaks to the respect with which Tim is held, as well as his role in leading a lifelong pursuit to be the best partner possible in the quest to improve outcomes for mothers and babies in Ghana and beyond.

When Tim Johnson talks about Ghana, his face lights up, his speech quickens, and the air in the room begins to feel charged. This book is the next best thing to being in the room when Tim starts talking about Ghana. With vivid descriptions and prose that puts the reader "in the room," this book provides an in-depth look at one of the most remarkable movements in global maternal health in our time: Tim Johnson's relentless drive to create sustainable, mutually beneficial partnerships to improve outcomes for mothers and babies in Ghana and around the world.

More Than "First, Do No Harm": Academic Global Health captures the heartbreaking drivers that led Tim Johnson to spend his career addressing maternal mortality in Ghana, at the same timing paying homage to the amazing, lifelong friendships and partnerships that have resulted. This book lays bare the key ingredients for sustainable, lasting academic partnerships in global health.

—Cheryl A. Moyer, MPH, PhD
Associate Professor of Learning Health Sciences and OB/GYN
Associate Chair of Diversity, Equity and Inclusion
Associate Director, Global REACH
University of Michigan Medical School

The approaches to Global Health that emerge from this story should transform Global Health development activities from traditional vertical programing to a commitment of building in-country capacity for comprehensive maternal and women's health improvements. Dr. Johnson has shown that a complex and committed effort to develop high quality academic obstetrics and gynecology programs transform the health system, enriches the academic lives of faculty and students in both countries and have a long-term multiplicative effect improving quality of life and survival.

Current "5 year" and problem-focused global health activities will never achieve the transformational results from the "academic partnership" approach described in this book. This book is a wakeup call to the Global Health Development community to program long term academic partnerships for a sustained, effective and self-growing health care improvements. Besides increasing the retention of Obstetricians in country, and thousands of lives saved, countless other jobs and new facilities and national leaders have been created. This program has had an incredible impact on the economy of Ghana—a multi layered impact that no single global health initiative could ever claim.

The approaches to global health development that emerge from this book are a blueprint for academics who want to sustainably contribute to health improvements throughout the world. The potential to end preventable maternal mortality starts when a country has the capacity to deal with the most complicated obstetric emergencies. Without academic institutions to create the modern obstetric care capacity in the many places where it does not exist, the goal will not be achieved. The amazing results from this project must be replicated to achieve the end to preventable maternal mortality.

The ethical assumptions that emerge from the stories shared by Dr. Johnson are health equity and justice through long term academic partnerships implemented with respect and evidence-based medicine. Only by building the full capacity to create and maintain modern obstetric capacity will preventable maternal mortality be eliminated. The amazing stories in this book come together reveal lessons that provide a blueprint for the elimination of preventable maternal mortality worldwide.

—Frank W.J. Anderson MD MPH, Professor and Chair,
Department of Humanities, Health and Society,
Herbert Wertheim College of Medicine,
Florida International University

More Than "First, Do No Harm"

More Than "First, Do No Harm"

Academic Global Health

Timothy R. B. Johnson

Edited by

Bradley R. Johnson

Maize Books

Published in the United States of America by
Michigan Publishing
Manufactured in the United States of America

DOI: https://doi.org/10.3998/mpub.12669456

ISBN 978-1-60785-762-4 (paper)
ISBN 978-1-60785-764-8 (e-book)
ISBN 978-1-60785-764-8 (open-access)

An imprint of Michigan Publishing, Maize Books serves the publishing
needs of the University of Michigan community by making high-quality
scholarship widely available in print and online. It represents a new model
for authors seeking to share their work within and beyond the academy,
offering streamlined selection, production, and distribution processes. Maize
Books is intended as a complement to more formal modes of publication in
a wide range of disciplinary areas.

http://www.maizebooks.org

Back cover: Mary Sue Coleman, President of the University of Michigan,
arriving in Kumasi, Ghana where she was met by UM alumni during her
groundbreaking trip to Sub-Saharan Africa. (courtesy: Ray Silverman).

To my family and my teachers

Pregnancy-related deaths are often the ultimate tragic outcome of the cumulative denial of women's human rights. Women are not dying because of untreatable disease. They are dying because societies have yet to make the decision that their lives are worth saving. Simply put, they die because they do not count.

Mahmoud Fathalla, MD

Chance favors the prepared mind.

Louis Pasteur

My experience can be summed up in four words: knowledge, sweat, inspiration, opportunity.

Yuan Longping, Chinese (rice) plant scientist

Nature is not a very good obstetrician.

J. Robert Willson, MD

I got to treat and I got to train to treat, what more can one ask for?

George W. Morley, MD

Those who stay will be champions.

Bo Schembechler, legendary Michigan football coach

You can't think yourself into a new way of acting; you have to act yourself into a new way of thinking.

Larry Bossidy and Ram Charan, in
Execution: The Discipline of Getting Things Done

Contents

Abbreviations

ACOG	American College of Obstetricians and Gynecologists
AMC	Academic medical centers
APGO	Association of Professors of Gynecology and Obstetrics (United States)
CREOG	Council on Resident Education in Obstetrics and Gynecology (United States)
FHMS	Family Health Medical School (Teshie, Accra, Ghana) at FHH (Family Health Hospital), part of Family Health University College (FHUC)
FIGO	International Federation of Gynecology and Obstetrics
GCPS	Ghana College of Physicians and Surgeons
GPTP	Ghana Postgraduate Training Programme (in Obstetrics and Gynaecology)
HOD	Head of department = chair equivalent in Ghana
JHIEPGO	Johns Hopkins International Education Program in Gynecology and Obstetrics
KATH	Komfo Anokye Teaching Hospital (Kumasi)
KBTH	Korle Bu Teaching Hospital (Accra)
KNUST	Kwame Nkrumah University of Science and Technology (Kumasi)
LMIC	Low- and middle-income countries

MCH	Maternal and child health
MCQ	Multiple-choice question (test questions)
MDG	Millennium Development Goals (UN) 2000–2015
MFM	Maternal-fetal medicine
MOH	Ministry of Health
OBGYN, OBSTGYNAE	Obstetrics and gynecology
PNDC	Provisional National Defence Council (Ghana)
RCOG	Royal College of Obstetricians and Gynaecologists (London)
RHFP	Reproductive health and family planning
SDG	Sustainable Development Goals (UN) 2015–2030
SMS	School of Medical Sciences (KNUST and UCC)
SOGOG	Society of Obstetricians and Gynaecologists of Ghana
SPHMMC	St. Paul's Hospital Millennium Medical College (Ethiopia)
TNBC	Triple-negative breast cancer
UDS	University for Development Sciences (Tamale, Ghana)
UGMS	University of Ghana Medical School (Accra, Ghana)
UHAS	University of Health and Allied Sciences (Medical School Ho, Volta Region, Ghana)
UM	University of Michigan
UMHS	University of Michigan Health System
USAID	United States Agency for International Development
USUHS	Uniformed Services University of the Health Sciences
V-C	Vice-chancellor
WACS	West African College of Surgeons (Ibadan, Nigeria)

Glossary of Terms

1. Basic science research: Often called "bench research," this is research performed in a lab (hence the bench) using basic science techniques or non-human models (molecular, cellular, animal, or theoretic models).
2. Translational research: Often called "bench to bedside," this takes basic science research or discoveries to clinical applications and practice.
3. Randomized controlled trial (RCT): This is a type of scientific experiment that aims to reduce certain sources of bias by randomly allocating subjects to two or more groups (experimental vs. control) and then comparing them with a measured response. The control group receives an alternative treatment, preferably a placebo, or sometimes no intervention. The trial may be blinded, meaning that information that may influence the participants and the observers is withheld until after the experiment is complete. A blind can be imposed on any participant in an experiment, including subjects, researchers, technicians, data analysts, and evaluators. The randomness in the assignment of subjects reduces bias in the assignment of treatments. Blinding reduces other forms of subject and experimenter bias.
4. Health services research (sometimes called "outcomes research"): Health services research studies outcomes of care, results of surgery or other interventions, quality, and safety. It also evaluates programs and policies.

5. <u>Implementation science</u>:   Implementation science promotes the uptake of research findings into routine health care in both clinical and policy contexts.

6. <u>Implementation engineering</u>:   Implementation engineering promotes the uptake of research findings and design science into routine health care (or other fields) in clinical, supply-chain, and policy contexts.

7. <u>Design science</u>:   Design science studies the creation of artifacts and systems and their embedding in our physical, virtual, psychological, economic, and social environment.

Acknowledgments

How does one go about acknowledging the people (much less the events and places) that played important roles in my over thirty-five-year affair with Ghana? My wonderful parents introduced me to the world when, as very young child, they took me with them to Yugoslavia, where my father was deputy air force attaché at the US embassy in Belgrade. All the people in our house, from a beloved nanny, Annie; Frau Maria, the cook; and a handyman, whom I later learned was a Soviet observer planted in our house, spoke Serbian, which I learned better than I knew English. I am sure this is one of the reasons I have had some subsequent facility with language and phonemes. During those three years, we reportedly traveled around Europe, and one of my earliest memories was being present in London for the coronation of Queen Elizabeth; from that I think comes my fascination with country flags.

Back in Virginia, for one of my father's many postings at the Pentagon, I started first grade at age five, and Miss Smithers was the first of many adored Nellie Custis Elementary School teachers. In 1963 we moved to Stockholm, Sweden, with my younger sister, Missy, and I started ninth grade (*quatrième*) at L'École Française, as there was no American or anglophone school in Stockholm. I had wonderful teachers in small classes at the French School; Mlles. Sirantoine and Carrier were among the French nuns who directed the school with a cloister on one of the upper floors of the city center school building. I still remember fondly (mostly) M. Davin, M. LeCovec, Mme. Hellman, and other teachers who came to our classroom, since there were only eight to ten students in my entire class from the ninth to eleventh grades in Sweden. The nuns were very tolerant of the coed French-taught international students who formed a separate cohort from the all-girl Swedish section, which had recently been attended by the royal Swedish princesses. Even in mid-1960s Europe/Sweden, we were exposed to progressive social mores: condoms were stocked in the boy's bathrooms. It seemed very tolerant and adult, especially by the time we got to eleventh grade. Returning to the United States, a plan to complete high school in Arlington altered after we had arrived there, and my father's military orders changed from the Pentagon to Scott Air Force Base in Illinois, where I spent the last year at Mascoutah Community High School. My credits from Sweden meant that all I needed to pass in my senior year to graduate was gym, which I hated, almost failed (and I continue to hate all things exercise), and that added to my adolescent anger at being in the middle of rural Illinois. Wonderful teachers—Mrs. Van Aiken in English and Debate, Mrs. Cunningham in Latin—and a few classmates, especially the members of the debate team, including Eva Jefferson (Patterson), made the year memorable (that's one word for it; it was 1967 after all), and soon I was off to Michigan for a wonderful undergraduate experience. Theodore V. Buttrey, chair of Classics, who taught Great Books; Martin Schwarz, who taught Junior Honors French (which I took as a freshman); Martin Stiles, chair of Chemistry, who taught Organic Chemistry; and magnificent French professors Floyd F. Gray, Jean Carduner, and Michel Guggenheim, who directed a unique summer graduate program in Avignon under the auspices of Bryn Mawr College, were truly memorable teachers and made my undergraduate and graduate years rich and meaningful. Many college friends who remained meaningfully lifelong friends include Larry Meisel, Leonard Gross, Warren Brauer, Dennis Plautz, Dan McMurtrie, and Bob and Victoria Buckler. By 1971, I had an AB (bachelor of arts) degree with distinction and high honors, an AM (master of arts) degree (both in French), an air force ROTC commission, and I was on my way to medical school. I surprised myself when I was accepted at all five schools I applied to: Michigan, Medical College of Virginia, University of Virginia, Georgetown, and George Washington. I wanted a smaller medical school class size and a less rigid structure (Michigan had a quiz every Monday for the first two years), and I chose to try a new adventure and new horizons by going to Charlottesville. This decision was made before I met my future wife, Jo Denal Wiese, in March of my last year at Michigan, and that led to some "distance challenges," which we overcame.

First-year medical school was challenging following the November 1971 death of Jo's father, Bob Wiese, in a plane crash on his way to a Michigan football game that I simultaneously was driving to, with Jo awaiting our arrival in Ann Arbor. We married in 1972 and Jo finished her Michigan degree in 1973. As I write this, we have been married for fifty years.

My second year of medical school was more enjoyable, especially pharmacology, where I had Al Gilman, MD PhD, and Ferid Murad, MD PhD, as lecturers, with no thought that these clearly bright, engaging junior faculty who forced us to absorb lectures about their seemingly obscure research topics, G proteins and nitric oxide signaling, would go on to win Nobel Prizes for their work. Doctors Edward Hook, William Muller, Norman Thornton, Peyton Taylor, and Siva Thiagarajah were excellent clinical and academic medical role models, both personally and professionally. It was as a second-year medical student that I was introduced to research through an extended nine-month research elective, this time at Wayne County General Hospital, affiliated with the University of Michigan, where I was introduced to men and women who would hugely influence my career: Doctors William C. Witting, Russ Laros, John Gosling, Mel Barclay, Alan Compton, Bruce Work, Bob Jaffe, and the department chair, J. Robert Willson, who would subsequently be my department chair as a resident. Not only were these doctors excellent clinicians, but they also excelled in medical education, Doctor Willson as an author of medical texts and as a leader in obstetric medical education. (He was a founder and president of the Association of Professors of Gynecology and Obstetrics, APGO, which would be central to much of my career and where I served as president forty years later.)

My early introduction to clinical research included my introduction to Joyce Mercer, a clinical research nurse, who taught me respect and admiration for nursing colleagues as partners and teachers. This continued into fellowship with nurse specialist, and later midwife, Trish Payne, and it continued in lifelong partnerships with nursing leaders like Barb Dubler, Liz Bole, Sue Kofflin, Carolyn Sampselle, Carol Boyd, and fabulous midwives including Lisa Paine, Carolyn Gegor, Terri Murtland, Trish Crane, Joanne Bailey, Holly Power, Lisa Kane Low, and many more at Michigan and in the American College of Nurse-Midwives. After medical school, I was deferred by the air force to complete residency in obstetrics and gynecology, and then fellowship. Doctor Willson and Doctors Jan Schneider, George Nolan, George Morley, John Gosling, David Anderson, Judith Pagano, Ivan Pelegrina, Lydia Prado, S. J. Behrman, Pete Peterson, and numerous coresidents became my teachers. Fellowship followed at Johns Hopkins with Doctors John W. C. Johnson, Jennifer Niebyl, my cofellows Norm Daikoku, Victor Khouzami, and other faculty, like Doctors Ted King, Ron Burkman (who would "invite" me to Ghana years later), and many cofellows and resident colleagues: Frank Witter, Howard Zacur, and John Repke all played important roles in my development as a maternal-fetal specialist and—equally importantly—as a medical educator. During my air force and Hopkins years and subsequently at Michigan, I had so many dear and influential mentors and colleagues: Doctors Edward Wallach and J. Donald Woodruff, who were important department leaders, role models, and mentors, and Doctors Peter Dans, Ed Goldberg, Phil Urso, Bill Hoskins, Iffath Hoskins, Tom Peng, Mike Gallagher, Joe Wax, Mary Jo Johnson, Terry Feng, C. D. Hsu, Ron Thomas, Tony Sciscione, Brian Iriye, Eva Pressman, Karin Blakemore, Bernie Guyer, and Janet DiPietro. Back at Michigan as chair in 1993, I got to be a colleague of my teacher George Morley, and on my first day as chair, Doctor Willson called from retirement in New Mexico to wish me well. In retrospect, the stories I had heard during training from Doctor Morley about his work in Brazil, Doctor Willson about his work in Germany after World War II restoring the academic OBGYN department in West Germany under the auspices of the Unitarian Service Committee, and Jack Johnson's stories about his time spent teaching at University College Hospital in Ibadan, Nigeria (where John Lawson, whom I was to meet later in Ghana, had been the first department chair), all probably created a unconscious backstory to what would become my Ghana experience.

Mark Pearlman (my closest administrative partner for many years), Frank Anderson (who most closely partnered with me and shared in my global health interests), John Delancey, Cosmas Vandeven, Clark Nugent, Bob Hayashi, John Randolph, Yolanda Smith, Dee Fenner, Kevin Reynolds, Carolyn Johnston, Margaret Punch, Lise Quint, Lisa Harris, Vanessa Dalton, Senait Fisseha, Maya Hammoud, Jason Bell, Ed Goldman, Lucie Moravia, D'Angela Pitts, Kayte Spector-Bagdady, and Emma Lawrence, our first Global Women's Health Fellow, were among the many faculty members who joined to make the UM OBGYN department great. The department was full of people who were great partners and team members, led for my entire tenure as chair by Jane Juckno, my executive assistant and "hand of the chair," Denise Fleming, Pam Stout, Janet Hall, Jennifer Edwards, Jennifer Jones, and Carrie Barroso. Other major colleagues at Michigan over the years who have been critical to my success include colleague chairs Tachi Yamada, Lazar Greenfield, Bob Kelch, Valerie Castle, Chuck Krause, Carol Bradford, Kevin Tremper, Reed Dunnick, John Greden, Greg Dalack, Bill Barsan, Paul Lee, Philip Zazove, my close friend and colleague/collaborator, family medicine chair Tom Schwenk, and former hospital president John Forsythe, who along with Giles Bole gave me my most important and satisfying job ever. Regents from Phil Power, who wrote to welcome me before I ever left Hopkins, to Andrea Fischer Newman, Mark Bernstein, and Rachel Bendit; university presidents Lee Bollinger, Mary Sue Coleman, and Mark Schlissel; and medical school deans Giles Bole, Allen Lichter, and Jim Woolliscroft were important in many successful programs and policies. Many people outside the department were great colleagues and partners: Pat Warner, Robin Menin, Lori Carpentier, Lloyd Jacobs, Joel Howell, Reshma Jagsi, Joe Kolars (director of Global

REACH and dean for global initiatives), Cheryl Moyer, Kofi Gyan, Andrew Boakye, Gurpreet Rana, Ray De Vries, Kelly Askew, Ray Silverman, Sabaratnam Arulkumaran, Clare Last Addington, Harold Kaminetzky, Denis Mukwege (a third important personal hero along with Mahmoud Fathalla and Allan Rosenfield), Abby Stewart, Marvin Parnes, Dan McMurtrie, Bob and Victoria Buckler, Jonathan Ayers, Rick Boothman, Irv Leon, Jean-Paul Pegeron, Mary Rumman, Shaun Maazza, Lee Tilson, Sue and Carl VanAppledorn, and Elaine and Peter Schweitzer have all helped me make my way. Nationally, former students have become important leaders, Andy Satin at Hopkins, and Chris Zahn and Maureen Phipps at the American College of Obstetricians and Gynecologists. I thank my friend Bert Peterson, distinguished global reproductive and public health leader at University of North Carolina, for writing the foreword to this book. He has been a major proponent of implementation science in the global context, and I think the Ghana project has been a poster-child project for this new discipline.

In Ghana, Jack Sciarra, Tom Elkins, John Lawson, John MacVicar, Adetokunbo Lucas, Patricia Rosenfield, and E. Q. Achampong, as well as J. O. Martey, J. B. Wilson, C. A. Klufio, Paul Nyame, Jacob Plange-Rhule, Peter Donkor, Seth Ayettey, Richard Adanu, Yao Kwawukume, Kwabena Danso, Emmanuel and Renée Morhe, and Joseph Seffah, along with many, many other Ghana medical school faculty, were all foundational and instrumental in making and keeping the Ghana program successful. Like all the people I have mentioned, and failed to mention, their influence on me and their importance to the events described in this book are immeasurable, and I can never recognize or thank them enough. Their wise leadership and management and their excellence as medical educators will forever be unsurpassed in my mind.

This is only the first example of many names and lists of names you will see me write about in this book. This represents how important individuals are in education, especially graduate medical education. People matter, teachers matter, individuals really make a difference, and their impact is lifelong and meaningful. Usually this impact is positive, but we all learn occasionally by negative example. I am sure I have, but I don't remember or recognize those names (except for my high school gym teacher). I have included many names in this narrative to emphasize the importance of many individuals in the success of the Ghana Postgraduate Training Programme in Obstetrics and Gynaecology, or GPTP (Ghanaians use British spellings). Those who do global health work need to remember that their success will always be dependent on and measured by the individual partners, learners, and others who participate in their initiatives.

Special thanks to my family, which has all my love, my parents Myra and Tim, my sister Missy (Myra), my wife Jo and children Brad, Clark, and Anna, and their families: Lauren, Emma, and Dylan; Brook, Timothy, Penelope, and Piper; and Danny and Lucy (so far). Their sacrifices and support have made my work in Ghana possible. I thank all these people and the many more not mentioned on whose shoulders I have stood and who have taught and supported me on my path. We have done this work together; this is a story of my teachers and my family, and for my teachers and my family.

Foreword

Herbert B. Peterson, MD, FACOG

With the launch of the United Nations (UN) Sustainable Development Goals in 2015, we had the first-ever commitment of world leaders to the health and well-being of each and every person on the planet. This vitally important moment in human history comes with both immense opportunities and challenges—achieving this unprecedented goal will require not only the "will" to do it but also the "way" to do it. Science has much to contribute on the latter front, including enabling us to continuously improve our ability to generate lifesaving and life-enhancing interventions—particularly those designed to be highly effective in low- and middle-income countries, where far too much of the global burden of disease and disability remains. Further, science, including the new and rapidly evolving field of implementation science, can help us to reduce these unacceptable health disparities by assuring the equitable, successful, and sustainable implementation of these interventions at scale.

I have had the great privilege of knowing the author of this important book—an esteemed academic obstetrician/gynecologist and giant in global women's health, for decades—and I share his passion for the contributions that the academy can make toward achieving health and well-being for all, particularly with regard to building scalable and sustainable capacity for implementing global health solutions. In this regard, I likewise share Tim Johnson's optimism that implementation science has the potential to make vitally important contributions toward achieving this goal and greatly appreciate the examples he so ably provides of realizing some of this potential.

Dr. Johnson's vision for the role of academe in global health and his clarion call for realizing the potential for this role began, as he describes at the outset of his book, with his experience of seeing more maternal deaths at a Ghanaian hospital in one night than would occur over decades in his own institution. The experience of the striking inequities between the risk of pregnancy and childbirth in the United States and Ghana—where, as he notes, a common phrase is "Pregnancy is a long journey and many women do not return"—led him to envision the Carnegie Ghana Postgraduate Training Programme in Obstetrics and Gynaecology. The Programme, funded by a grant to the University of Michigan from the Carnegie Corporation of New York in 1989, is a truly exemplary indication of the potential for academe's contributions toward building sustainable capacity for promoting health and well-being in low- and middle-income countries—and a blueprint for helping to achieve it. By 1995, the Programme was being sustained by the Ghanaian government and by 2017, had trained 246 specialists in obstetrics and gynecology—nearly all of whom had stayed to practice in Ghana or were practicing in the African subregion.

The success of the Programme—which, as Professor Johnson notes, emphasizes the importance of local context, as well as leadership and engagement at the local level—is all the more remarkable in that it has provided a roadmap for replication elsewhere. As he describes, the Programme was reproduced successfully in Ethiopia in just four years, as opposed to the initial eight in Ghana—based largely on lessons learned from the Ghanaian experience. Further, the program in obstetrics and gynecology was replicable to multiple other medical and surgical disciplines in Ghana's two medical schools, with counterpart programs being launched in emergency medicine, family medicine, otolaryngology, ophthalmology, and psychiatry, among others.

We are living in a moment filled with great promise—one in which we have recognized unacceptable disparities in global health and committed to addressing them. Realizing this commitment will require making progress not only in the contributions of our great universities to the generation of lifesaving and life-enhancing interventions but also to their implementation equitably, successfully, and sustainably at scale. This book, written by a renowned academic who has "walked the walk," is as inspiring as it is informative with regard to realizing the potential of the academy to do just that.

Herbert B. Peterson, MD, FACOG
Kenan Distinguished Professor
Department of Maternal and Child Health,
Gillings School of Global Public Health
Department of Obstetrics and Gynecology, School of Medicine
Director, WHO Collaborating Centre for Research
Evidence for Sexual and Reproductive Health
University of North Carolina at Chapel Hill

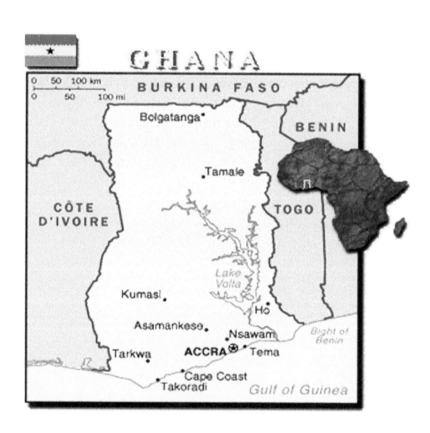

CHAPTER 1

Introduction and
the "End of the Story"

In 1989, the Carnegie Corporation of New York funded a grant to begin the training of specialist obstetrician/gynecologists at the teaching hospitals of Ghana's two medical schools: Korle Bu Teaching Hospital, at the University of Ghana in Accra, and Komfo Anokye Teaching Hospital (KATH), at the Kwame Nkrumah University of Science and Technology (KNUST) in Kumasi. As of summer 2017, 246 specialists had been trained and virtually all stayed to practice in their country or the African subregion ($n = 236$, 6 have died in Ghana, 3 came for training from the Gambia and returned to their country to practice, and 1 emigrated to the United States with his American wife [Kekulawala et al., 2022]). The program is now self-sustaining and, since 1995, has received support from the Ghanaian Ministry of Health, Ministry of Education, and the Ghana Health Service (Anderson et al., 2007; Clinton et al., 2010). Since 1993, robust programs in emergency medicine (Martel et al., 2014; Mould-Millman et al., 2015; Osei-Ampofo et al., 2013, 2018; Oteng and Donkor, 2014; Oteng et al., 2020), family medicine (Essuman et al., 2019; Toma et al., 2020) otolaryngology (Waller et al., 2017), ophthalmology (Global REACH, 2019), psychiatry (Natala, et al., 2018), and other medical disciplines (Essuman, et al., 2019) have evolved at these same teaching hospitals, all with the involvement of University of Michigan Medical School faculty. Medical student exchanges going in both directions remain established, as well as exchanges of residents (medical school graduates who are pursing training as specialists in areas such as surgery, internal medicine, or obstetrics/gynecology, called "postgraduate trainees" or "postgraduates" for short in Ghana, and "resident," "house officer," or "graduate medical education (GME) trainee" in the United States; "intern" is no longer formally accepted for those in their first year of residency, although widely used) (Abedini et al., 2014, 2015; Danso-Bamfo et al., 2017; Lawrence et al., 2020). Numerous faculty and nurses at various levels have also been exchanged. The University of Michigan Medical School's Global REACH office became very active in coordinating robust global health activities in a small number of countries, designated as "platforms," and eventually the greater university and its presidents, Mary Sue Coleman and, subsequently, Mark Schlissel (Chapter 11), became involved as these platform programs extended broadly to include hundreds of undergraduate, graduate, and professional students working in interdisciplinary, intergenerational, and often interprofessional teams. Operational and programmatic lessons from the Ghana experience have been broadly adopted in schools and colleges across the university. Presidents Coleman and Schlissel have both highlighted the Ghana experience and model as they have publicly spoken about institutional goals, aspirations, and values in academic global education. In a one-on-one discussion with him, President Schlissel asked me: "How did the Ghana program and your involvement start?" One of my goals and purposes in this book is to tell the story of how and why the Ghana Postgraduate Training Programme in Obstetrics and Gynaecology (GPTP) started. But more importantly, I hope to offer a blueprint and "lessons learned" from the Ghana program's university-wide expansion, with a strong suggestion that these can be generalizable and implemented, modified, and transformed at and between other academic institutions in the United States, other countries, and across continents. The critical key attributes demonstrating the valuing of local culture, context, and true local participatory engagement and leadership will hopefully be continuously in view. That must truly be the prime directive. Most importantly, I hope that student learners, faculty and others interested in engaging or enhancing their engagement in global health, and academic global engagement writ large, who read this book will carefully consider their personal involvement and institutional programmatic development, as well as a variety of critical clinical, behavioral, and ethical underpinnings for the practice of truly engaged and principled academic global health.

Chapter 2

"But for..."

In 1986, I had just finished four years of military payback at the air force teaching hospitals and had joined the faculty of Johns Hopkins Hospital as an assistant professor of obstetrics and gynecology. My particular task was to develop a "fetal assessment center" to evaluate the health and well-being of high-risk fetuses. I was busy building a career in maternal-fetal medicine (MFM), a medical subspecialty covering high-risk obstetrics formally established in the 1970s. At the time, I was doing many invasive prenatal tests, such as amniocentesis, complex deliveries, and counseling, and eventually did the first percutaneous umbilical blood sampling (PUBS) at Hopkins—a new invasive test where ultrasound is used to sample blood from the umbilical cord. I had done my fellowship in MFM at Hopkins from 1979 to 1981 following an obstetrics and gynecology residency at the University of Michigan. I had developed substantial interest in public health, especially disease prevention for women, prenatal care, and maternal mortality and morbidity, but global and international health was not on my radar, nor did it form any significant part of my previous medical education or training experiences.

Hopkins had an international program, the Johns Hopkins International Education Program in Gynecology and Obstetrics (JHIEPGO), founded by Doctor Theodore "Ted" King, the director of the Department of Gynecology and Obstetrics (Hopkins fashioned a flip of the usual disciplinary designation). King, a truly visionary global health leader, initially developed JHIEPGO to take advantage of developing laparoscopic technology to perform and disseminate female sterilization and assist with population control. This was an early example for me that technology often drives programmatic innovation. Family planning is what funders—both the United States Agency for International Development (USAID) and private foundations—were interested in in the 1970s, but by the mid-1980s, JHIEPGO grants supported international faculty development, educational programs on sexually transmitted diseases (STDs), reproductive health, family planning, contraception, and other similar programs across the globe. I interacted with and often taught classes to the faculty from international institutions and departments who came to Baltimore for JHIEPGO courses. Initially embedded in the department, JHIEPGO subsequently moved toward independence, first situated in the School of Public Health, and then, as subsequent department heads became less interested in supporting the program with faculty being pulled from their financially important clinical activities to teach locally and globally, it moved to being administered by the Johns Hopkins University Office of the Provost. The large indirect costs that accompanied the grants were desirable financially to the university (see Chapter 11). Eventually, JHIEPGO became a free-standing non-governmental organization (NGO) with few ties to Gynecology and Obstetrics or other academic units, except that Hopkins medical school faculty who were interested in global health could and would continue to participate in the local and international programs as instructors. It even dropped "Johns Hopkins" from its name and continues to operate under its acronym alone.

Doctor Ronald Burkman was one of those faculty members deeply engaged in education and training globally through JHIEPGO. He was an associate professor in the Department of Gynecology and Obstetrics with interests in family planning and contraceptive technology. He had an international reputation for his extensive research on efficacy and safety of intrauterine devices, before they were in fashion, and he went on to become department chair at Henry Ford Hospital in Detroit, Michigan, where our paths were to cross again. The reader will become aware, as I have, that academic obstetrics and gynecology, and academic global health as well, are "a small world."

In mid-1986, Doctor Burkman stopped by my Hopkins office to inquire whether I might be interested in a JHIEPGO-sponsored trip to Ghana. He was supposed to give a presentation to the Society of Obstetricians and Gynaecologists of Ghana (SOGOG) on family planning, contraception, and a laparoscopy update, but he found himself unable to go. I was interested, but his planned presentation topics were not really my areas of expertise. I suggested presenting on prenatal care, medical complications of pregnancy, and advances in maternal-fetal medicine, and he was fine with that. I had a few months to prepare, get a visa, passport, yellow fever shot, and get my "slides" together. This was pre-PowerPoint, and I had files of photographic slides I used to prepare lectures. Fortuitously, JHIEPGO was holding an advanced faculty development course in Baltimore during the time before my departure, and a young faculty member from the University of Ghana Medical School, of similar junior rank to me, Doctor A. B. Amoa, was in attendance. We had a chance to meet, he filled me in a little on Ghana, and I was happy that there would be a contact I would know in Ghana during my stay.

The purpose of the Ghana meeting was to reestablish, with a national medical conference and banquet, the Society of Obstetricians and Gynaecologists of Ghana, which had lain fallow without meeting for over a decade during the military regime of Flight Lieutenant Jerry Rawlings and the Provisional National Defence Council (PNDC) government, which had seized power violently for a second time in 1981. Until the mid-1980s this totalitarian Ghana government had been "eastward looking," with support mostly from the Soviet Union, its satellites, and Cuba. By 1986 the Iron Curtain was coming down, the disintegrating USSR was reducing its support of satellite foreign governments, and the United States was becoming a dominant superpower, so Ghana was turning warily to the West for a new relationship. It was in this geopolitical context that my trip was arranged.

The Ghana OBGYN Society was going to have this first meeting in years, supported by USAID funds through JHIEPGO, and I was the featured guest speaker. An important highlight and draw for doctors from around the country was to be the well-attended "gala closing event" banquet—a typical professional society and organizational conference arrangement all around the world.

I arrived in Ghana, and at the time the Accra airport was primitive. Kotoka Airport, the site of a major military-political coup and bloody executions, was named after a famous military leader. The heat hit me as soon as the plane door opened, and the sweet, humid smell was one that I would come to recognize as the smell of the tropics. "Arrivals" was a thatch-and-grass-covered open-air hut at the side of the runway, and there was table after table of paperwork and bureaucracy. Everything was done by hand with pencils, pens, and numerous hand stamps on documents. The arrivals area was oppressively hot, and there certainly was no air conditioning, not even fans. After initial customs, there was passport control, then federal police control, then local police control, and then baggage was delivered in another outdoor space, followed by another several customs controls and a detailed baggage search. Outside the airport doors, masses of people crowded around, pulling at your luggage, hands out asking for help, offering to help find a taxi: to anyone used to US domestic travel it was chaos. Luckily, someone from USAID picked me out and took me to the US embassy guest house where I was booked to stay, since USAID was officially sponsoring my travel and the event. Even in 1986, I noted that the security at the guest house was tight. Uniformed guards took their time to examine the contents of the trunk and looked with large mirrors on wheels under the official car. The embassy guest house was an oasis with air conditioning, most importantly, and a comfortable room and bed in a walled compound with several security guards at all times. While there was finally air conditioning, in 1986 it went off every few hours during the day and night, and transformers would sometimes kick in and sometimes not.

I definitely had not brought appropriate clothes for the tropics, since I felt that, as a "Professor," I had to wear my usual button-down pressed shirt, bow tie, and blue blazer.

One of my first scheduled events after a night's rest at the US embassy guest house was attendance at morning report at the Korle Bu Teaching Hospital (KBTH) affiliated with the University of Ghana Medical School. This was held in a tightly packed, un-air-conditioned room in the hospital, and I sat in the front row. Little did I know how many dozens more times I would sit in the same room, usually in a suit and tie and in a front row, listening to reports and updates. But that morning report is one I have never forgotten. Morning report is a medical tradition around the world, and especially important in obstetrics, where there is action twenty-four hours a day. The purpose of morning report is to inform the clinical team coming on duty what happened to patients in the previous twelve to fourteen hours and what they might expect to encounter clinically when they take over clinical responsibility for the unit—in this case the labor and delivery and gynecology units. In addition to a traditional and formulaic litany of the patient's age, number of pregnancies, obstetric and medical condition and complications, morning report is also an opportunity for faculty and others to highlight clinical treatment, teach pathophysiology, develop plans of care for the patients on the unit, and make dispositions on surgical scheduling ("this woman needs a cesarean delivery right away," "this woman needs to have her labor induced") or therapy ("this woman needs antihypertensive therapy"). Most institutions do not have comprehensive clinical guidelines or pathways, and certainly these did not exist in Ghana in 1984, so clinical recommendations are often articulated "in the light of day" and going forward. Most institutions do not have faculty or specialists present overnight in the hospital, and certainly they were not present in KBTH, where even phone contact was difficult in 1986. Morning report can also serve as a teaching opportunity for house officers, interns, and medical students, and with over twelve thousand deliveries, this was certainly true at KBTH.

At my introductory morning report—and my introduction to clinical medicine in Ghana—the presenter, probably a chief resident, started

out by reporting that there had been ten maternal deaths the night
before. A faculty discussant then noted that there would be no way all
ten deaths could be discussed, so the presenter should present one or
two remarkable cases, or make some general comments about common
issues observed in the cases. Ten maternal deaths! I came from an institution where there was a maternal death about once every three to four
years, and here was something an incredible magnitude higher. I had
long read, and even written in book chapters, about the high maternal
mortality in low-income countries, but it was something else again to
come face-to-face with the reality. I don't even remember details of
the discussion after that. I do remember the repetition of the words
hemorrhage in labor, operative hemorrhage, postpartum hemorrhage—
hemorrhage, hemorrhage, always hemorrhage. And seizures, usually
seizures associated with a condition that obstetricians around the world
know well, preeclampsia, where hypertension in pregnancy, in ways
poorly understood, combines with kidney failure and brain swelling to
cause seizures and death. In the United States, an inexpensive therapy,
magnesium sulfate ($MgSO_4$) given intravenously, followed by delivery,
mitigates and prevents the seizures and prevents complications. But
in Ghana, the disease was not diagnosed soon enough, and with inadequate therapy and no access to $MgSO_4$, the clinicians saw seizures,
more seizures, and death. And finally, I heard about infection—*fever,
antibiotics, sepsis, and shock*—and death. Everywhere in the world,
hemorrhage, hypertensive diseases, and infection constitute the triad
of the most common causes of maternal mortality, but here in this
room at KBTH, the scale and scope of the problem were like nothing I had ever seen, and certainly my experience had not adequately
prepared me for something I had not really ever fully imagined. The
hour passed very quickly; only a very few patients and clinical teaching
"pearls" had time to be presented and discussed. After the conference,
I retired to tea in the HOD suite (head of department being equivalent to the department chair) and air-conditioned faculty offices across
the hall from the conference room. That is what always happens with
visiting "professors." Maternal mortality was a reality that I had been
aware of. I had acknowledged it in several chapters on prenatal care

that I had authored, and in 1986 it was the impetus for the international Safe Motherhood Initiative (Mahler, 1987; Maine & Rosenfield, 1999; Sai & Measham, 1992; Starrs, 2006; Tita et al., 2007), but it had always been presented to me and by me in traditional, medicalized fashion. It became real to me that morning, and I will never forget that initial Ghana morning report. But we are all visual learners, too. As we left the building, I walked down the marble steps of the maternity block with consultant specialist leaders of the OBGYN department. At the time it was a temporary maternity block, because as is often the case in Ghana, interminable work was being done on some part or another of the hospital. To the left of the main entrance of the hospital, next to the steps leading from the maternity block to the parking lot, was a flatbed truck with "Morgue" painted on the cab door. On the flatbed were ten bodies, still clothed in the bright blue, yellow, and red that all Ghanaian women were wearing, the clothes that they stayed in during childbirth and delivery at KBTH. These were the bodies of the dead from the night before. They were piled neatly and carefully. All dead, they displayed the bright colors of the clothing that I had seen on the streets and in the hospital halls and wards. Clothing that defined them as individuals, no longer in a medical or medicalized setting, but individuals who would not ever be returning to their families, their homes, or their lives.

Those bodies haunted me from that moment. They haunt me today—and as you will see, they also inspired and inspire me to action. They gave vivid color and reality to the burden of maternal mortality and the importance of the Safe Motherhood Initiative. They represented mortality that could have been prevented. My determination to make global health part of my life began at that moment. My resolve was reinforced when I heard later, maybe not on that visit but a later visit, that a commonly voiced Ghanaian saying was "Pregnancy is a long journey and many women do not return." That was totally inconsistent with how we think in the United States. We do not expect or even conceive that a woman might die when she enters the hospital for childbirth. On the contrary, maternal death is almost always thought of as a result of malpractice and a terrible error. I was further galvanized by the words of Professor Mahmoud Fathalla, an Egyptian OBGYN, former president of the International Federation of Gynecology and Obstetrics (FIGO), and an articulate visionary and champion for women, whom I had heard speak a call to action at a FIGO international meeting in Copenhagen: "Women are not dying of diseases we can't treat. They are dying because societies have yet to make the decision that their lives are worth saving." (Fathalla, 2006). Professor Allan Rosenfield, then dean of the School of Public Health at Columbia, had inspired the Safe Motherhood Initiative with his landmark 1985 paper in the prominent British journal the *Lancet,* titled "Maternal Mortality—a neglected tragedy. Where is the M in MCH?" (A. Rosenfield & Maine, 1985), detailing the lack of reduction of maternal mortality in low- and middle-income countries when at the same time a marked drop in neonatal (newborn and early childhood) deaths was being recorded. Fathalla and Rosenfield are two of my personal medical and reproductive health heroes.

I gave my prepared talks and they went fine, although the regular 2″ × 2″ slides in use at the time, pre-PowerPoint, needed special projectors, and most of the lectures at UGMS were given with old-style, large glass slides using old lantern projectors. Finding "modern projectors," much less having electricity available when needed, was an issue. The projectors obviously only worked when there was electricity, and it came on and went off regularly, so several of my talks were given with a blackboard and chalk—and I actually enjoyed the old-style lectures at the blackboard with chalk, in the old-style lecture halls, and the spontaneity of marshaling my thoughts and teaching priorities in this way.

I met most of the few active medical school OBGYN faculty: Doctor John Baptist "J. B." Wilson was the head of the Department of Obstetrics and Gynaecology; Doctor Amoa, whom I had met in Baltimore, was there, as was Doctor Armah, who was interested in OBGYN infections and would subsequently come to Hopkins to do an advanced clinical skills course (where we would further develop our relationship); and Doctor Ghosh, an Indian and British Commonwealth appointee (supported by UK funds), who had been in Ghana for several decades and was highly respected. Doctor Ghosh was a beloved physician and teacher who dedicated himself to his patients and his students. He never married. He was always asking clinical questions, especially of the medical students, and seeking answers in the medical literature, which at the time meant books, often old and out-of-date books. He was an amazing role model to all his students, including me. When his multidecade posting in Ghana by the British Commonwealth ended, he was returned to India where, we heard from a brother, he died shortly after his return. Truly a life dedicated to service. I came to find out he loaned books from his large collection—a very precious commodity—to medical students and housemen (undifferentiated postgraduates in the first year or two out of medical school), but mostly to young postgraduates who aspired to be obstetrician/gynecologists. Books continued to be a precious commodity during the first decades of the training program that was subsequently developed. Doctor Tom Elkins and I took seemingly endless trunks full of hardcover books with us on subsequent flights to Ghana, air baggage being more reliable, faster, and almost as cheap as shipping them. I remember vividly that they were incredible heavy and bulky to manage through airports, especially at "Arrivals" in the heat of the tropics. Once information became available on compact discs and smartphones, carrying books, having books, even reading books, became a thing of the past. I was so grateful when we could take the equivalent of many trunkloads of books over on a singly floppy disk or Zip disk.

In 1986 in Ghana, after medical school (seven years after high school) and a year or two (it varied with the policies or, more accurately, the whim of the Ministry of Health) of "housemanship" (equivalent to the old American rotating internship)—six months on medicine, pediatrics, obstetrics/gynecology, and surgery—young physicians could enter preliminary obstetrics and gynecology training. After two years minimum, and after a basic science exam followed by an initial written clinical exam (called "Part 1"), they would hope to get a post and financial support to complete formal training in the United Kingdom, Europe, or the United States. Doctor J. B. Wilson had trained in the United Kingdom, as had Doctor Amoa and most of the other Ghanaian OBGYN faculty, although some had trained in Germany or Russia, either for medical school, residency, or both. Doctor Ghosh had formally trained in India, and later at the SOGOG meeting I met Doctor J. O. Martey, professor and head of the department in Kumasi, who had done training in Manchester, England, a very famous department, home of the internationally well-known gynecologic surgical "Manchester procedure." Many Ghanaians had completed their medical school training in the United Kingdom before the University of Ghana Medical School opened in 1964; a few had trained in Ibadan in Nigeria. The most notable thing I heard and absorbed was that twenty-six doctors had left Ghana to do OBGYN training abroad with the support of the Ghanaian government, usually the Ministry of Health, and/or with financial support of the sponsoring countries, which were getting much-needed doctors to supplement their own staff doctors to provide patient care and other necessary services at the same time that they were getting training. None, NONE, of those twenty-six had returned to Ghana. Many were still in the United Kingdom, Europe, or the United States, where they had trained. Increasingly, younger, mid-career Ghanaian obstetrician/gynecologists who had trained abroad were serving in the Middle Eastern countries, where they were highly sought and highly compensated as OBGYN practitioners and consultants. A highly respected professor, Doctor Cecil Klufio, who had been groomed for OBGYN leadership at UGMS, was in Papua New Guinea with unclear hopes of when, if ever, he might return to teach students and young doctors. Doctor Amoa, my friend from Hopkins and the "Osu Castle adventure" (see Chapter 3), who had trained in the United Kingdom and received JHIEPGO/USAID–sponsored faculty development, soon joined him there, where he remains to this day. These were all well-paid jobs where these obstetricians could earn enough money to support themselves, their families, send their children to good schools (Doctor Klufio's daughters attended Wellesley and Stanford), and often, send funds back to their families in Ghana.

Everyone, especially the young doctors, wanted opportunities to train in the United Kingdom and the United States. Doctor Ghosh was loaning them books to read. Women were dying. One day while making rounds, I was presented the case of a woman with a congenital form of dwarfism called achondroplasia, who had presented to KBTH after laboring several days in her village. No one there had ever considered that she might (surely, as could have been expected) have difficulties in labor and delivery, and she presented to the hospital with a dead, undelivered baby requiring a cesarean section to save her life. As a result of the obstructed labor, she developed a vesicovaginal fistula, an opening between the bladder and vagina, caused by tissue necrosis and sloughing from the pressure of the dead fetus's head pushing against maternal tissue. The medical students were very interested in spending some time with me and arranged an extra clinic with "interesting" and complicated patients for the "professor from Johns Hopkins" to see with them. The patients presented to me that day by the medical students all had obstetrics fistulas from obstructed labor. They wondered how we managed these challenging cases at the famous Johns Hopkins Hospital. I had never in my career seen a traumatic obstetric fistula, much less a clinic full of patients with such fistulas. All the patients wanted help. All the medical students wanted to know how to help. One of the fistula sufferers was the sister of one of the medical students. It was unlikely any of these women would ever be able to obtain a surgical repair of their fistula, which would be curative. No resources. No clinical capacity. Not enough doctors. Not enough doctors with the special skill to repair genital tract fistulas. Everyone reminded me of the crush of people that first met me upon exiting the airport—hands out, desperate for help.

But these doctors and medical students I met were fantastic to be around. They were smart. They were book smart. They pored over and memorized the few old, precious, well-worn texts available to them. They were clinically smart. They were able to make a diagnosis by taking a careful, detailed history with their hands for palpation and their stethoscopes for auscultation, by looking under their patient's eyelids, and a few basic laboratory tests. They were really good clinicians. I saw them operate, and they were really good surgeons. They were deft and quick in surgery, and they did it all well with one suture and few critical instruments, in half the time and with a quarter of the suture material we used in the United States. They walked around with a packet of suture, some antibiotics, some basic lifesaving medications like oxytocin (to treat postpartum hemorrhage), and even local anesthetic solutions in their pockets—and they used them when the resources were not available in the hospital to save their patients' lives. In this context, cesarean delivery or surgery for ectopic pregnancy can be life-saving by preventing hemorrhage and infection. Operating rooms often did not function because there were no anesthetic gases or injectable anesthetics. Large empty gas canisters were standing in empty operating rooms. All surgery was done with local or spinal anesthetics. The doctors used their "personal stash" in the instant for emergencies, and then the patients' families had to go to the market, where antibiotics, anesthetics, suture, and bandages were all available for purchase. It often took families days to pull together the money, and their family member was not discharged from the hospital until the supplies were returned to the doctors to resupply their "stash."

If patients needed blood transfusions, the family had to go to the blood bank and make the donation. But that only happened during the day. The blood bank was closed at night, and therefore nothing available if a woman exsanguinated "after hours." The few anesthesiologists at the hospital were not available from five or six o'clock in the afternoon until the next morning. There was no overnight coverage. It was just how it was.

So I saw unimaginable clinical pathology; maternal deaths; smart, well-trained doctors; basic facilities overburdened with patients; occasional anesthetics; poor access to blood; medications; sutures; and limited access to operating rooms.

The SOGOG dinner was a success. It was catered in the cafeteria of the maternity block, across from the hospital and the doctors' parking lot. The few obstetrician/gynecologists from the community, the few UGMS faculty, and housemen and postgraduates were in attendance. Doctor Mary Grant, the PNDC (government) minister of health, came and we talked about the future with hope: the future of the society, the future of obstetrics and gynecology in Ghana. The Ghanaians I met were inspiring. The need and the potential of the future were clear. The opportunity at that moment in time was inspiring to me, not only in the context of the worldwide Safe Motherhood Initiative (Mahler, 1987) but also with the changing political winds in the country. A past department chair, Professor Ampofo, who had an MPH from Hopkins and had a vision of past success and glories, was there and spoke formally at the meeting, as did Doctor Grant. It was as if Ghana was emerging from a time warp of inactivity, a politically left-leaning military regime, a "closed-in" period that reminded me of Cuba's closed culture. In fact, Flight Lieutenant Rawlings, an avowed Socialist, had many dealings with Cuba, and Cuba sent many of its doctors to Ghana to practice, especially in the rural areas. It was a time of stasis, a time when every good initiative and effort to improve women's health was happening outside Ghana.

The gustatory highlight of the dinner was a huge grilled fish Ghanaians called "sea bass," a delicious food memory that would be joined by many more in the years to come. Much can happen within the fellowship of shared professional identity and good food. The attendees all got a certificate of attendance, and I was lucky enough to remember to ask for signatures from the group, a treasured souvenir of those in attendance and an important memento of who was there at the very beginning.

I returned to Hopkins overwhelmed by what I had seen, educated about the burden of maternal mortality. I guess I had a prepared mind, and I saw a need for more obstetrics and gynecology doctors to prevent and treat this burden of women's disease in Ghana. I really admired the doctor leaders, the faculty, and the young doctors I met. And I was an academic educator. I had been interested and involved with medical education since my own residency, when medical students gave teaching awards to the most involved residents. I had trained residents at Kessler Air Force Base, at the Uniformed Services University of the Health Sciences (USUHS), where I worked with family medicine residents, and then a maternal-fetal fellowship training program at Bethesda Naval Hospital. I was an academic physician who taught and trained people. Medical education was my comfort zone and my wheelhouse.

JHIEPGO was not really focused on postgraduate resident training at the time. It promoted skills training programs for practicing doctors and faculty development (see Chapter 7). I decided to pick up the phone and call the American College of Obstetricians and Gynecologists (ACOG). Let me interject that this was a big step for me. I am by nature an introvert, and very shy socially. I am sure this will surprise many people because I can be outspoken in a group and surely sometimes talk too much. I have always been reticent to use the phone to call people I don't know or don't know well, especially "important people." Calls to people I don't know well especially scare me. I am still working on this. Electronic messaging has been easier, but it can be a barrier to direct contact when it is needed. Self-confidence and appropriate assertiveness are learned attributes. The executive director of ACOG, Doctor Warren Pearse, an important and powerful person and senior leader in the OBGYN profession, was someone I knew and who knew me. He had done his OBGYN training at Michigan, had been chair at Nebraska, and dean at the Medical College of Virginia. He knew of my work improving prenatal care clinics and resident and medical student education at Hopkins. *I picked up the phone.* I took a chance to make a call. I took the chance to call Doctor Warren Pearse and asked him if ACOG ever supported training in Africa. I had come away with the idea that the thing to do was in-country OBGYN residency training in Ghana. Warren Pearse listened to my story about my trip to Ghana and the urgent need for more OBGYN physicians. "No," he said, ACOG and its training affiliate, the Council on Resident Education in Obstetrics and Gynecology (CREOG), did not have money for or experience in international resident training. But, Doctor Pearse said, it was a strange coincidence that I had called. Just the previous week he had hosted a personal visit from the new president of the Carnegie Corporation of New York, who had met with him at the ACOG offices in Washington to discuss an interest in CREOG capacity building and training, specifically in Africa, in the context of the Safe Motherhood Initiative. Doctor Adetokunbo Lucas, a renowned Nigerian-born and Harvard-trained public health physician, and a friend and colleague of Doctor Allan Rosenfield, the same OBGYN and Columbia School of Public Health dean who wrote about the "M in MCH," was newly ensconced as leader at the Carnegie Corporation of New York (Lucas, 2010). Doctor

Pearse gave me the contact information, and I picked up the phone and called Doctor Lucas. Yes, he was interested in health capacity building in Africa. Yes, he thought the idea of a residency program to fully train obstetricians and gynecologists in Ghana was good and potentially feasible. Yes, the Safe Motherhood Initiative and maternal mortality were interests of his, the concept was potentially fundable, and he would welcome a grant proposal. Full credit to Adetokunbo Lucas. It was as if he had been preparing for just such an opportunity for years, and he no doubt had. Even though he was trained in community medicine in Nigeria and had been department head in Ibadan, he understood primary, preventive health care and the principal components of women's health. No doubt the extended training he had as a medical student and house officer enhanced his experience base and understanding. And he was the consummate academician, a skilled politician, and a natural orator.

Several names came up in that initial conversation, including Doctor Tom Elkins, a global health expert working in Western Africa, along with a few others demonstrating the potential for broad interest and engagement. Doctor Lucas said he would entertain a proposal to fund an exploratory meeting on funding for OBGYN training in Ghana if there was support from ACOG in Washington, and the Royal College of Obstetricians and Gynaecologists (RCOG) in London, especially Lucas's old friend and obstetrics professor from Nigeria, Professor John Lawson. The idea of the Ghana Postgraduate Training Programme (GPTP) was conceived.

What drove my vision, which quickly became a shared vision, for an in-country training program? First, the global Safe Motherhood Initiative made improved maternity services to reduce maternal mortality an international priority. That was the message and the lesson of Doctor Allan Rosenfield and his "Where is the M in MCH?" call for action (Rosenfield & Maine, 1985). Second, I was a medical educator. I had been trained by well-recognized national leaders such as Doctor J. Robert Willson and Doctor George Morley (both former presidents of ACOG) at Michigan, and Doctors John W. C. "Jack" Johnson and Ted King at Hopkins, all of whom prioritized teaching medical students and residents. I had valued my own fellowship training with such mentors as Doctors Jack Johnson and Jennifer Niebyl. Jack spoke repeatedly and fondly about a memorable experience he had teaching for a few short months in Ibadan, Nigeria, but I never listened very closely, never understood the possibility that such an experience could be indelibly meaningful, and never considered that I would ever visit, must less work in Africa. I had embraced medical student education as a resident at Michigan and received a prized "Bronze Beeper Award" from graduating medical students. This continued at Hopkins, where resident education was added to the repertoire, and this interest continued in the military at Biloxi Air Force Base Medical Center in Biloxi, Mississippi, and then Andrews Air Force Base near Washington DC, where I was on the faculty of the USUHS and interacted with family medicine and OBGYN residents as well as medical students across multiple teaching hospitals in the National Capitol Region. One of the students who worked with me for several weeks at Andrews, Andy Satin, is now the Gynecology and Obstetrics (backwards as always) department director (chair equivalent, a contrarian designation as always) at Johns Hopkins. I received medical student and resident teaching awards on numerous occasions during this time (including the J. Donald Woodruff Award from the Hopkins residents, named after one of my most influential teachers). At Hopkins, when I returned there to the faculty in 1985, I was shortly appointed as the OBGYN residency program director, so education was "what I did," and it should not be surprising that I was able to see the opportunity for academic resident training in Ghana. And finally, it was clear from what I knew in 1986 that the doors to opportunity for training for African doctors were closing in the United Kingdom and United States, especially for OBGYN and surgical training, where there was huge rising demand from their own growing domestic crop of graduating young doctors. The Ghanaians who had been waiting patiently doing junior doctor rotations over and over with poor pay, providing services to patients, and allowing consultants to work in their private offices were not ever going to get specialist training as they had dreamed. This soon became an issue, since early program candidates and trainees thought the GPTP was going to prevent them from leaving for training, and they were vociferous and angry in their opposition to the program. John Lawson and I were to have several very uncomfortable meetings with a few of these older but still "junior" doctors, and it required real control to accept their aggressive and assaultive language. John learned some American techniques of civility from me, and I some British and Nigerian tricks from him. It was a good thing for him that I was in some of those meetings, and I will talk about some of the lessons of Sir William Osler and his famous essay "Aequanimitas" (Sokol, 2007), which probably informed my tendency to stay calm and cool under pressure, in the next chapter. The only way that OBGYN training was going to be available in the near term for Ghana was a local program. A local program would teach local diseases and local practices much better than US and UK programs, where malaria and obstructed labor were unlikely to exist and, I thought, would better prepare doctors to practice in their country. This turned out to be true, and it also turned out to be a major factor in the extraordinarily high in-country retention that we would achieve throughout the years of the program.

It was also at this point that I had to decide how this global work was going to fit into my life. I was a busy academic. I was getting more responsibility as residency director, fellowship director, and division chief. I had to worry about publications and promotion. And my life included a young family. In 1986, my children Bradley, Clark, and Anna were nine, five, and one. I wanted to work in Ghana with new colleagues and friends, and new teaching and organizational challenges (I guess I liked and was good at working in complex health systems. "Health system" is now one of the competencies we are required to teach our medical students and residents, but it was not identified in the explicit or even implicit curriculum at the time), but I could not stretch myself too thin. Today it is recognized and called "work-life balance." I decided to work just with Ghana. JHIEPGO has projects in many African countries, Southeast Asia, and the Indian subcontinent. ACOG and RCOG had interests in many countries. I was going to do Ghana. Just Ghana. It proved to be the right strategy for me. And a strategy I regularly recommend to others.

What is the point of this chapter? What are the takeaway messages? What are the lessons for those thinking to forge a global program and a global career? Remember that this whole story started with a call from a colleague asking if I wanted to give some lectures. What was different about this call from Doctor Ron Burkman was that the lectures were in Ghana. Perhaps I will remember to ask him why he called me when I see him again. The important point is that **but for** that phone call, I and my prepared mind would not have traveled to Accra, and I would not have had the transformative experience I have described so far. I would not have conceived of some of the initial programmatic possibilities. I decided to make some phone calls. Basically, cold calls. I was a busy clinician, back from a week away, jet-lagged, and with lots to catch up with. I picked up the phone. **But for** the call to Doctor Warren Pearse, I would not have connected with Professor Lucas. **But for** the visit to ACOG from Lucas, his interest and that of the Carnegie Corporation of New York in the Safe Motherhood Initiative would not have been known to Doctor Pearse. **But for** the concurrent timing of the international Safe Motherhood Initiative, the shared vision would not have coalesced. For me, the important lessons were: 1) just do it, and 2) don't procrastinate. If the opportunity presents itself, if the door appears, grab the handle and go through. If an idea or a vision develops, follow though and "pick up the phone." The metaphor should be clear: go for it. And as I learned from my mother: do it now.

Lessons Learned

When the door appears, open it.
When you have an idea: Just pick up the phone. Do it now.
People matter. Individual action matters.
Opportunity can precede vision, and vice versa.
Focus on <u>one country</u>. Make long-term personal connections there.

CHAPTER 3

"Despite…"

Not everything went smoothly with that first trip. JHIEPGO had regular courses on faculty career development and various other reproductive health topics in Baltimore, and there was enough time between Ron Burkman's invitation and the trip to Ghana that I was able to meet a Ghanaian physician who was in Baltimore for a JHIEPGO course. Doctor A. B. Amoa was a young faculty member in OBGYN at UGMS. He was friendly, personable, and a very well-trained and knowledgeable obstetrician/gynecologist whom I was able to meet and talk with before my departure. His JHIEPGO course timing was such that he would be back in Ghana by the time I arrived. Actually, his time in Ghana was going to be limited, as he and his family were moving to Papua New Guinea, where he was joining a senior respected Ghanaian obstetrician/gynecologist professor. I would later find out this was Professor Klufio, whom I would meet when he returned to Ghana and became a director of the GPTP. He would become a good friend and authored the first peer-reviewed report on the GPTP (Klufio et al., 2003), which he also presented orally at the Association of Professors of Gynecology and Obstetrics (APGO). Two important principles supported by all involved evolved organically early in the days of the program, which

I embraced from the onset of the collaborations and continue to embrace: 1) always involve local authors in research and publications from the onset, and 2) PUBLISH the reports of innovative educational programs in peer-reviewed journals (yes, publish or perish pertains everywhere). So both Doctor Amoa and Professor Klufio, who were either in or moving to Papua New Guinea in 1986, were actually part of the brain drain that I had already heard about, and continued to hear so much about.

I was able to reconnect with Doctor Amoa in Accra, and the pre-arrival contact was very helpful in making us feel comfortable with each other. He was personable, clearly a skilled clinician, and very well prepared to be an academic and clinical teacher. Evident in Baltimore, this was even more evident watching his interactions with colleagues and postgraduates in Korle Bu Teaching Hospital.

One of the perks that set more senior doctors apart from juniors was a good car, and Doctor Amoa had a Volvo. We had one afternoon free, and he drove me around to "see the sights," one of which was the Osu Castle, an impressive white structure near the ocean that had been built as a slave castle by the Dutch. It was the presidential residence of Flight Lieutenant Jerry John Rawlings, and we drove around chatting animatedly about stuff that colleagues talk about. This was the time of the military government of the PNDC, the Provisional National Defence Council, Rawlings's second post-coup government, which had been in power for about five years. The transition away from a paranoid military rule that began with a bloody coup and the execution of many previous military and political leaders at the Teshie barracks firing range (close to the sites of the Kofi Annan International Peacekeeping Training Centre and the Family Health Medical School, FHMS, which we will talk more about later) had only just begun. As we were driving around to get a good look at the impressive and important white structure, suddenly our car was surrounded by uniformed men with handguns, submachine guns, and even more impressive shoulder-slung automatic weapons. We had been distracted by our conversation and driven past probably several "Do Not Proceed Past This Point" signs and got "too close!!" to restricted space. A car with a black driver with a white face in the passenger seat clearly raised suspicions, and more armed men surrounded us and the car, with the apparent leaders repeatedly asking why we were there and why we had ignored the signs. Soon the military guards were joined by men in civilian clothes with impressive handguns in their shoulder holsters and in their hands, clearly "secret police," and we were told to leave the car and follow them. We followed them closer to and then into the "castle" through guarded barriers and doors into an open central courtyard. The courtyard was large and filled with tanks. The tanks were arranged so that the gun barrels were aimed at the gates and doors that gave access to the presidential "palace," clearly pointing to points of potential ingress and prepared to respond to any attempt to storm the castle.

At that point, Doctor Amoa and I were separated, and I was led down two flights of stairs to a sub-basement, where I was placed in a room with a table and chair. My passport was taken from me, and I was given a pencil and legal pad and told to write down how I got there and who I was. I remember seeing several clearly new, brightly colored anti-AIDS campaign posters, one with prominent condoms and penises with a clear warning directed to the security guards and men of the castle to encourage safe sex. I was encouraged (remember this was 1986, the early days of the AIDS epidemic, before effective treatments) and glad that even two floors down in the bowels of the presidential palace, guards were getting the message to use condoms—and avoid "loose women." I was not so glad that I was in the sub-basement of the palace, having seen some imposing "internal security measures," without my passport and with no one anywhere in the world having any idea of where I was. I calmly thought that I would probably not get out alive, that I would simply disappear, never to be heard of again—and I say "calmly" because what could I do? I was surprised at my calmness in the face of an unknown fate that I had no control over. I think my experience in calmly dealing with obstetric emergencies (that I had no control over) and the calming exhortations of Sir William Osler (one of the famous four founding doctors at Johns Hopkins and the first professor of internal medicine) in "Aequanimitas" (Sokol, 2007), his reflections on a proper attitudinal approach to medicine that are quoted endlessly at Hopkins, were key to my lack of fear and anxiety in the situation. It was a medicalized state of mind I had learned to use while watching over patients in labor, while waiting for anesthesiologists to induce anesthesia, while operating on women with obstetric complications, while sitting in stressful administrative and academic meetings. I was surprised by my "equanimity" at the time, and I remain surprised by it more than thirty years later. I had, however, been implicitly trained by my teachers, and my experiences, not to panic in clinical situations. And that carried over to academics and almost every other situation. When things got out of control with patients, emotions, or families, or there was major bleeding or difficulty extracting a baby, I was trained to be calm, to be the adult and the leader in the room (the captain of the ship, the choreographer, the conductor of the orchestra and all that). I had learned from both negative examples and positive role models how to deal with clinical stress, and it carried over into this personal situation. I waited and waited, having written everything I could think of on the yellow legal pad with the pencil I had been given.

After what turned out to be almost three hours, a man in civilian clothes, and with impressive, shiny black handguns at his hips and shoulder, said to follow him up the two dark, narrow flights of the old slave castle to the ground floor and sunlight, where I was reunited with Doctor Amoa, and we were taken together by car to the central police station. We drove past his car, which appeared to have been nearly dismantled with panels off the doors and all the seats removed. I never heard if he ever got his car back. Neither of us had a camera—I suspect that is what the authorities were looking for—and if they had found one, I truly believe both of us would have disappeared in Osu Castle, never to be heard from again. The formality of the Accra central police station made me feel safe. We were met by very tall, imposing, and very professional officers in black uniforms. I still feel more at ease when I see Ghana police officers in their impressive black uniforms.

We were in-processed, which meant our names were inscribed in large books that looked like something the long-suffering Bob Cratchit from *A Christmas Carol* would have used. We also had our passports handed back and, as we were still in suits and ties, were handled with some degree of careful attention. We were placed in a large cell with a dirt floor—a floor that reminded me of the floors of the slave castles I had visited previously—a constant reminder of the many people who had been in those cells before. Sweat and desquamated skin cells stained the floor and scented the air. The other detainees all seemed to be shirtless and shoeless, in either short pants or loin cloths, and they eyed us with both disdain and interest.

That was the scary political situation in 1986. Rawlings subsequently transitioned to a civilian dictatorship, then to an elected civilian government, during which he famously welcomed Bill Clinton to Ghana (Clinton Avenue still exists near the airport) and, in a remarkable moment of statesmanship, handed the reins of government to an opposition party when they won the next election. I was honored to meet Rawlings (now deceased) in 2016 at the opening of the FHMS, which would be founded by one of the residents we were about to train in the nascent GPTP.

I have subsequently come to find out that there was reason for the Ghanaians to worry about American faces in 1986. USAID, and even JHIEPGO, I have come to believe, often had CIA or similar intelligence operatives embedded in or accompanying their program participants in countries around the world. The USAID programs, whether food programs or health sector/academic development, were the perfect cover for United States operatives interested in information. My father's long-time military service had been with the National Security Agency, Defense Intelligence Agency, and Air Force Intelligence Agency. During our time in Stockholm in the 1960s, where he was the air and defense attaché, our travel often included flights on a US military–marked embassy plane that flew between Sweden and West Germany, often "straying" very close to, if not over, parts of East Germany. When we spoke shortly before his death, when he was sharing more from his past, Dad was surprised I had not been aware of the many cameras in the undercarriage of the embassy plane. I should have been more situationally aware of this, but I guess even in 1986 I did not put it together.

We were told by the Ghana police that the US consular office would be contacted to arrange bail, if they would pay it. Eventually, an American consular officer came and paid 1,400,000 cedis (yes, one million, four hundred thousand cedis), about ten dollars in the rapid Ghanaian 1986 inflationary spiral, and we were released to his care. I was told I needed to report each day to the central police headquarters until the matter was settled. The next day, "Madame X" (I never got her name), a uniformed, very official-looking policewoman sitting at a desk in front of piles and piles of "Scrooge's ledger books," added my name to one of them and then told me I would have to report back to her to have my name recorded in her ledger every day. It was clear no one would ever be able to find anything among all the piles of bureaucratic filings. (Just as was often true, I would come to find, in the medical records of the Ghanaian teaching hospitals.) When I asked her how long I would have to do this and when I would be cleared, she shrugged. This was a problem, since I was supposed to leave Ghana just a few short days after the "Osu Palace" adventures. When I asked a consular officer and the people at the United States guest house what I should do, they shrugged. On day three after my arrest, I signed in with the chatty, friendly, but officious "Madame X" in the afternoon, went to the airport, and boarded my Swiss Air flight. I worried that I would be pulled off the flight, but as I had hoped, paper ledgers did not provide the tracking of even 1986 computers. No one really cared about me and my offense, and I breathed an air-conditioned sigh of relief when the plane took off into the dark night from Accra's Kotoka Airport. Now it is a wholly modern international airport, with the main building in the shape of a Ghanaian stool—a very impressive edifice both when arriving and departing. No more thatched roofs. In 1986, looking out the windows after takeoff, most of the lights were from cooking fires. Today, airport departure is over the lights of a modern city until several miles out, when the brush and cooking campfires reappear with an occasional modern TV screen as visual human signals of change from the ground to the thoroughly modern jet.

Doctor Amoa went to Papua New Guinea in 1986 and remains there still. People hope he will come back on faculty in Ghana, like Professor Klufio did. I understand that the educational opportunities for his children are a major factor in his decision to stay. And I bet by now it's his grandchildren's education. Professor Klufio's work in Papua New Guinea was able to support his daughters, who went to Wellesley and Stanford. He lives with them in the United States, now in retirement.

Despite the "near-death" experience at Osu Castle (and the fear that "Madame X" might actually be able to track me down), I never hesitated to return to Ghana. Now we laugh about the storied and oft-repeated experience, and Osu Castle is an interesting museum open to the public. The tanks are gone. Ghana has benefited from political and economic stability, and from repeated peaceful presidential regime changes and transfers of political power. Political and economic stability have been a hallmark of Ghana's steady move from low-income to near-middle-income status. I have come to admire the peaceful transition of political leadership and power as one of the most important measures of modern democracy. Finding offshore oil didn't hurt either. All that has been essential for the continuing success of the Ghana Postgraduate Training Programme.

Lessons Learned

Global health engagement can present challenging, scary, even dangerous experiences.

Stay safe. Stay calm. Be prepared.

Resilience and persistence are necessary and required.

Do not give up your dream or your passion.

CHAPTER 4

The Carnegie Grant and Early Years

Adetokunbo Lucas (his memoir is well worth reading, see Lucas 2010) of the Carnegie Corporation of New York decided he wanted RCOG and ACOG engagement in the development of the grant proposal. RCOG offered John Lawson—an old friend of Lucas, vice president of RCOG, and a true African pioneer. After residency in Britain, Lawson went to the University of Ibadan to become head of the first OBGYN department in West Africa at the first teaching hospital, University College Hospital. Lawson was joined by Professor John MacVicar, an avuncular Scot who came from Professor Ian Donald's remarkable department in Glasgow, the home of obstetric ultrasound and leader in advanced perinatal ultrasound (which I related to professionally at Hopkins), where he had risen from trainee to Head of Department. Selected to represent the United States in addition to me were Doctor Jack Sciarra, long-time distinguished chair of OBGYN at Northwestern, a past president of FIGO, and editor of the International Journal of Gynecology and Obstetrics; and Doctor Tom Elkins, a gynecologist at the University of Michigan, where I had trained as a resident before going to Hopkins for fellowship. Elkins was very involved in African initiatives, mostly mission work in Nigeria, Ghana, and other countries. As the most junior of the participants, and out of interest in his own career advancement, Elkins was to write the formal grant proposal. There was to be heavy involvement by the Ghana Ministry of Health (MOH) , the Ghana Management Committee and the External Advisory Board. This language was very important as the Ghanaians were to be empowered to develop and manage their program, and the US and British roles were to be advisory. The Ghana Management Committee members were decided upon (J. B. Wilson, J. O. Martey, E. Q. Archampong, K. K. Korsah, and representatives from the MOH and from the Ghana Health Service, including Doctor Ken Sagoe).

The proposal planning for the grant required an initial meeting in London, in historic wood-paneled, stained glass–windowed rooms of the RCOG, which was attended by J. B. Wilson (Accra), J. O. Martey (Kumasi), a representative from the MOH, Jack Sciarra, Tom Elkins, Adetokunbo Lucas, John Lawson, John MacVicar, and me. At this meeting, the curricula and program requirements of the American College of Obstetricians and Gynecologists, the Royal College of Obstetricians and Gynaecologists, the American Board of Obstetrics and Gynecology, and the West African College of Surgeons (WACS) and their policies and processes were all discussed in detail. The desire for residency training in Ghana was endorsed by all, and the Ghanaians developed a program of what they wanted to achieve in Ghana that was consistent and fully aligned with WACS requirements. This required an entrance examination for acceptance into the program and an initial basic science examination soon after entry, which was very different from American examinations that required no such intense pretraining and testing in basic science, and even the RCOG was moving away from such rigorous initial basic science training. The entrance exams were to be taken after the candidates had spent one or two years practicing in regional hospitals, and significant review and study of basic science material would be required to pass these qualifying examinations. A proposal to send teachers with basic science expertise, mostly British since the British system required more basic science as part of their training, was planned to prepare Ghanaian candidates for the basic science examination.

The planned GPTP curriculum was designed to assiduously prepare trainees for two WACS examinations: a written Part 1 clinical examination and a final Part 2 examination at the completion of year 5, which consisted of both a written multiple-choice question (MCQ) and essay portion, and an oral examination that included evaluations of live patients (the "viva") and a case list that included two long commentaries (twenty to thirty pages, one in obstetrics and one in gynecology) and thirty short commentaries (three to five pages). An innovative program element was required community experience of six months, where the fourth-year (and therefore experienced) trainees would spend time in a community hospital without direct daily supervision. Instead, the faculty consultants would visit them on-site in the community hospital on a regular basis as they collected their cases. It was anticipated they would learn how to run a basic obstetrics and gynecology service, and by this time, before the fifth and final year, they would have enough experience to be able to do cesarean sections, cesarean hysterectomies, simple hysterectomies, myomectomies, and other common procedures, including dilatation and curettage. If they identified complicated cases, they could save them to be performed with the consultant faculty at the time of their site visits. In addition, during this community service time they would collect data for a required community-based research project. The thought was that community-based projects that used a preventive medicine approach would be popular, very useful to the candidates in the future, and probably publishable or at least hypothesis-generating for further research. This turned out to be true, and the community postings remain a unique and successful component of OBGYN training in Ghana.

It was also a requirement that the residents would take a full-time class at the Ghana Institute for Management and Public Administration (GIMPA) at the University of Ghana, which offered a twelve-week course that was commonly given for the mid-level public health sector trainees and others involved with public health policy and government service. It was to be offered to these relatively more junior obstetrician/gynecologists so that they would learn to work collaboratively and do interprofessional work, and thus be able to understand health systems and be change agents and leaders in the future more fully. Many of the Ghana faculty in Accra and Kumasi stated that they wished they had taken or could take the course. It was a very popular feature of the GPTP, and this is an offering and best practice that could well be implemented in domestic training in the United States.

There were further exploratory meetings in Ghana, with stays in the dean's guest house conveniently located a few short blocks from the Korle Bu Teaching Hospital compound but also only a block away from the hospital morgue. The screened windows had long since disintegrated, and I returned from one of my early Ghana trips to Hopkins and began feeling unwell. I developed a fever and chills, which I ascribed to the flu, but eventually developed severe headaches and an altered mental status. I had taken malaria prophylaxis, and it never occurred to me, but an excellent Hopkins infectious disease expert diagnosed cerebral malaria. I had the dubious honor of being presented as an "interesting case" to the weekly, always very well attended, Saturday morning internal medicine grand rounds. It was a "viva," a live presentation that not many Hopkins faculty got to participate in from the patient side. Apparently, the dean's guest house shared mosquitos with the morgue, and malaria was still common in Ghana. I wish I had a more complete recollection of what must have been a very erudite discussion of my condition, prognosis, and recommended therapy. I recovered completely, have never had a recurrence, and still am very compulsive about malaria prophylaxis whenever I travel to the Ghana and other endemic regions.

The dusty roads of the KBTH compound have been paved and the signs brightened since the 1980s, and the dean's guest house and nearby tennis courts have been completely modernized with excellent window screens. They have not moved the morgue (Asediba, 2022).

This program proposal was agreed to, further funding was secured, and the residency program was rolled out at a large celebratory meeting at KBTH in 1989, attended by the Ghana Management Committee, the External Advisory Board, and many, many interested residents.

An initial challenge concerned ensuring there were adequate faculty to teach in the program. In Kumasi, Professor Martey had an adequate

CV and was already appointed as a professor at KNUST. Doctor J. B. Wilson was an instructor, and the *most senior extant faculty member, Cecil Klufio, his presumptive predecessor and* later successor, and the next-in-line academic, Doctor Amoa, had both gone to Papua New Guinea to positions that were attractive both professionally and financially. This caused some leadership challenges, and attempts were made by the Americans and British, including meeting with the dean and a letter-writing campaign, to get the University of Ghana to consider Doctor Wilson's significant administrative and service contributions for promotion to assistant professor. To its credit, however, the university held firm to its criteria for promotion. The GPTP was overseen administratively (including the chair of the Ghana Management Committee) initially by Doctor K. K. Korsah, who was a retired senior doctor highly regarded by all, and subsequently by Professor Cecil Klufio upon his return from Papua New Guinea. Professor Klufio presented the first report on the successful program to the Association of Professors of Gynecology and Obstetrics and was first author on the first publication report on the program (Klufio et al., 2003).

There were additional challenges associated with the structure of the early years, mostly related to communication and interpersonal differences. There was a particularly high degree of contentiousness among the External Advisory Board members, specifically the British, and especially between John Lawson, who was a great clinician, an experienced academic and administrator, and an outspoken, unapologetic socialist (and supporter of the National Health Service), and Tom Elkins, also an excellent clinician and gynecologic surgeon with a big heart, who was also a religious fundamentalist with missionary zeal. John Lawson was a fascinating character who, as has been mentioned, had gone to Nigeria right after his residency in the United Kingdom and set up the first obstetrics and gynecology residency training program at the University of Ibadan in Nigeria. He became the first professor of the department and then went on to become the provost and vice-chancellor for a period of time. He told many terrific stories about his work during that time, including climbing behind his heavy desk during the shelling of the university during the Biafran War. His best and most instructive story to me was of his insistence, during the construction of the University College Hospital in Ibadan, that there be a swimming pool. Apparently, every time he put a swimming pool into the design plans it was crossed out. In the end, he executed plans for a large, adjacent "water containment and storage facility" that was approved, and he had his swimming pool. I have used a similar trick a few times. Part of his story is in his paper "The Bight of Benin and Beyond" in Appendix 2.

Lawson trained a generation of obstetrician/gynecologists and knew Adetokunbo Lucas from Ibadan, where Lucas had, in early days, been one of the founders of the Department of Community Medicine at the University of Ibadan. This relationship between Lawson and Lucas was probably important in the early years ,with both agreeing to participate and ensure that things went well. Professor John MacVicar, as I have said, came from Glasgow, the home of clinical ultrasound. He collaborated closely with and was a good friend of Tom Brown, the civil engineer with expertise in the use of ultrasound to assess the integrity and safety of large cement industrial structures, who used this vast technical engineering knowledge to assist Professors Ian Donald and John MacVicar develop the clinical application of ultrasound in obstetrics. Remember, my academic base at Hopkins was in fetal assessment, with ultrasound as an indispensable tool. Many years later, when I received an honorary fellowship from the Royal College of Obstetricians and Gynaecologists, Professor MacVicar was in the robing room accompanying Mr. Brown, who was recognized for his contributions with a long-overdue honorary fellowship at the same ceremony. I was very humbled to even be in the same cohort as this remarkable engineer who was there in the earliest days of the development of clinical ultrasound. Another "but for" event that would not have happened if I had not gone down a global health path.

One of the biggest lessons for me about doing health-related work in Ghana, and elsewhere in LMIC, came thanks to John Lawson: the critical importance of engaging and working with the MOH. I was used to working within university structures, but having spent years in Nigeria and in the United Kingdom, Lawson understood the importance of ministries in the successful function of universities and teaching hospitals. Lawson was able to bring together the US and UK advisors with the Ghanaian medical representative and Ghana's MOH, which was not an institution that I had any similar prior experience with. In the US, universities function autonomously, but in LMIC, the MOH is a key player in funding, programs, and policy. Ghana medical schools and teaching hospitals were dependent on the MOH for manpower and funding, so MOH representatives clearly had to be at the table. That lesson was invaluable for the success and sustainability of the GPTP and will remain an important theme in this story: success, sustainability, and reproducibility in LMIC require the input of academic institutions and Ministries of Health, and sometimes even Ministries of Education.

The hard and long part was making GPTP work. At the regular meeting that occurred about every six months in the initial years of the grant, usually in Ghana, the United States was represented by Thomas Elkins, John Sciarra, and me. The United Kingdom was represented by John Lawson and John MacVicar. For Ghana, there was J. O. Martey, J. B. Wilson, and Professor E. Q. Archampong, a famous surgeon and the University of Ghana Medical School dean, "blessed with a charming disposition and exemplary character" ("Emmanuel Quaye Archampong," 2023), and the representatives from the MOH, who varied and exhibited the most turnover (as government entities do). Turnover in government is more frequent than in the academy—another reason it is smart to pursue primary engagement with the universities to ensure program sustainability and assist in academic capacity building to ensure human capacity building.

The United Kingdom sent lecturers for basic science and Part 1 exam preparation. The United States sent clinical teachers. Lectures and slides were left behind so Ghanaians could use them in their role as teachers and professors. Education encompassed the introduction of curriculum and pedagogy, the expansion of clinical education, and the embrace of clinical research. This went on for the first three to four years of the program as the local Ghana pipeline began to fill with postgraduates. There were occasional disagreements and difficult meetings, but Ghanaians, as the Ghana Management Committee, always got the last word, although sometimes they had to gently give reminders and be insistent with the External Advisory Board. The universities were careful during this time to maintain their academic standards and waited until the initial GPTP graduates had the bona fides for appointment and promotion in the medical school. Dean and Professor Archampong saw to that. And it did not take long for professors to rise from within the program.

A major source of tension was between Tom Elkins, who, as a Southern Baptist evangelical, was committed to a whole series of unassociated missionary activities and initiatives. His language, attitude, and proselytizing infuriated the vociferous socialist John Lawson and annoyed John MacVicar, and the two of them were continually concerned about the issues and tone that Tom Elkins brought as chair of the External Advisory Board. Since Elkins had written the grant, this position had been given to him by default.

Doctor Elkins often went up to Nalerigu and cities in northern Ghana and even Nigeria to pursue his missionary work. He was very committed to these activities and had been working in Africa and Nigeria doing Baptist mission work for several years at this point. On one occasion, during a trip by Doctor Elkins with Doctor Jack Sciarra to some northern villages, an event occurred that will demonstrate some of the issues. Tom had scheduled surgery on some difficult fistula cases in a local Baptist hospital. One of the patients traveled to the hospital, staying locally, and Doctor Elkins met with her in preparation for surgery. He said to his companions that he wanted to do a pelvic examination on the woman and needed to find instruments and lighting. The more senior and serious Doctor Sciarra asked him not to do the exam that evening, but rather to wait until a more appropriate time to do it in a clinical setting before surgery. Everyone went to bed, but Doctor Sciarra was awakened and asked to go immediately to the clinic where Doctor Elkins needed him. Upon arrival, Doctor Elkins was preparing to operate on the woman. He had decided to examine her with flashlights and candles, and unfortunately the vaginal speculum had penetrated past the scarring of the fistula and the patient's scarred vagina had opened and bowel contents spilled out into and out of her vagina. Emergency surgery had to be performed to replace the bowel contents in the abdomen and close the top of the vagina. He should have listened to Doctor Sciarra. It required some extra hands and Doctor Sciarra was not happy to be operating in those conditions through much of the night before the planned early morning departure. I suspect that such stories were part of the reason that I never developed Tom Elkins's missionary zeal. Lawson, no doubt given his Nigerian experience and his subsequent UK academic and RCOG experiences, was very committed to institution building, capacity building, and academic growth, and he disdained missionary work both because of the religious aspects (he was devoutly atheist) and the lack of resultant sustainable human capacity building. As vice president of the Royal College of Obstetricians and Gynaecologists, he was very involved with its global activities and globalization, and his position gave him access to valuable RCOG resources. We were happy to make use of the comfortable RCOG facilities available for some GPTP Ghana Management Committee and External Advisory Board meetings in London since it was midway between Ghana and the United States. Lawson was particularly renowned and widely respected in the African subregion because of his reputation from Ibadan in Nigeria and because of his formidable book *Obstetrics and Gynaecology in the Tropics and Developing Countries*, published in 1967 (Lawson & Stewart, 1967). This had long been the definitive and only book on obstetrics and gynecology in the tropics until the Ghanaians were inspired to publish their own landmark books, *Comprehensive Obstetrics in the Tropics* in 2002 and *Comprehensive Gynaecology in the Tropics* in 2005, and a textbook on reproductive health (Kwawukume & Emuveyan, 2002, 2005; Olatunbosun, 2002). I invited Doctor John Lawson to give the inaugural endowed Nicholson J. Eastman Lectures at Johns Hopkins, in honor of a famous former chief of obstetrics there, and he talked about his experience with Doctor Eastman. In inspiring terms, he described an early visit to Baltimore to meet and visit with Doctor Eastman, who had spent several years at Peking Union Medical School in China, where he studied the use of magnesium sulfate for the management of pre-eclampsia. Lawson gave a brilliant talk entitled "The Bight of Benin and

Beyond" (Lawson, 1991; see Appendix 2), including comments about the influence that Eastman had on him before he set off to establish the Obstetrics and Gynecology Department in Nigeria, one of the many, many coincidences and profoundly and personally important events that happened during the course of my Ghana experience.

One last Sciarra story. During his trip to northern Ghana visiting several clinics, hospitals, and villages, Professor Sciarra, always meticulously dressed and with abundant and always well-coifed white hair, was the guest of honor at a great feast one evening at one of his stops. After abundant food and always terrific Ghanaian beer, Doctor Sciarra was horrified when the village chieftain offered him one of his daughters to marry (and probably also take back to America, to the significant benefit of her family and village). He demurred repeatedly and managed to leave with only the gifts that the chieftain absolutely demanded that he take: a goat and several chickens. Jack told me he simply could not get away without taking them. He also received a ceremonial headdress of feathers and beads that he described as fabulous. He left the village with headdress and animals among the luggage, and the inhabitants at the village that was the next stop were extremely happy with the lavish gifts they received from Doctor Sciarra: a goat, some chickens, and an impressive ceremonial headdress. I learned a lot about diplomacy at every level—from academic to global—from Jack Sciarra, and he remains an esteemed friend and lifelong mentor.

Elkins continued to annoy Lawson with his missionary activities, as well as with what was considered micromanagement by the British. Finally, Lawson and MacVicar met with me and Jack Sciarra and said that if Elkins remained as chair of the External Advisory Board, the RCOG would withdraw from the program. One of my first experiences giving people bad news was having to take Tom Elkins for a long walk and explain to him why his position as chair of the External Advisory Board would be taken over by Doctor Jack Sciarra, who, as the most senior of the ACOG representatives, an experienced department chair, and former president of FIGO, was always situationally aware and astutely diplomatic in all his interactions. Again, one of the things I learned from my Ghana experience was the difficult job of leaders giving colleagues and friends feedback and bad news. Subsequently, despite many philosophical differences, Tom and I talked a lot about issues, and shortly after he moved from Michigan to Louisiana, I moved to Michigan from Hopkins in an interesting series of musical chairs. He was very helpful in introducing me virtually and preparing me to work with the Michigan faculty and help them achieve success. Doctors Elisabeth Quint, Hope Haefner, and Margaret Punch were all assistant professors and went on to become professors during my time at Michigan, and Tom and I had spoken extensively about their career development plans at the dean's guest house in Accra. Faculty development is a continuous process that is demonstrably, once again, both opportunistic and intentional (Chapter 7).

Once Jack Sciarra took over leading the twice-yearly External Advisory Board meetings, which were no longer contentious, we slowly started to see progress through the program in both Accra and Kumasi. Doctor Kwabena Danso, who was Professor J. O. Martey's protégé and whom he wanted to see move quickly through the training to a faculty position, did his requisite community project at a regional hospital in Mampong Ashanti, completed excellent community-based research, and prepared for the Part 2 oral examinations. The first GPTP trainee who was successful in passing the FWACS exam in Ibadan was Doctor Addo Tagoe from Accra (now deceased); Doctor Yao Kwawukume from Accra was the second successful trainee to take the examinations. Doctor Danso followed the next year. All of them had spent time at Johns Hopkins, doing either academic development courses or STD/family planning courses as part of JHIEPGO, so I knew them from both the US side and the Ghana side. In fact, I was in Ibadan as an external examiner for the examination when Doctor Kwabena Danso passed the exam, wearing a confident smile and his Hopkins tie for good luck. Once the program started to be successful, the Ghana Management Committee was given substantial leeway, and they largely managed the grant to its completion in 1995. The total grant from the Carnegie Corporation was about $6 million, including administrative support, and was overseen carefully by Adetokunbo Lucas and the Carnegie program officer, Patricia Rosenfield (P. Rosenfield

2014). It covered travel for outside faculty to and from Ghana, travel of Ghanaian residents and faculty to and from foreign training and career development sites (mostly in the United Kingdom and United States), and meetings of the Ghana Management Committee and the External Advisory Board.

The initial years of the program were so successful in the production of OBGYN doctors who stayed in Ghana that the MOH took over the in-country training costs when Carnegie funding expired. External travel for all concerned then became dependent on other sources of funding. Based on the remarkable number of specialists trained and remaining in-country, the subsequent reverse brain drain of Ghanaian expatriates returning to practice in Ghana, and the broad replication of the program in other disciplines and in other countries, I have heard from colleagues at the Carnegie Corporation that the GPTP is considered one of the most successful programs in its history. The value proposition, the dollar-for-dollar return on investment, was high, and the program continues to produce a "return on investment." Unfortunately, the Michigan side of the grant had not been administered carefully, and one of my challenges moving to Michigan was to resolve financial issues with the Carnegie grant and "close out the grant." Funds transfers to Ghana and other global sites continued to be a challenge despite subcontracts and largely due to US university bureaucracy. It took until the Center for Reproductive Health Training was established under the direction of Doctor Fisseha (see Chapter 10) for financial transfers to be facilitated, and now most grants go directly to Ghana, Ethiopia, Rwanda, and other African partners. After 1993, given the financially confusing situation, it took several years for me to convince medical school leadership that global health programs were worth the effort, and they came around when they became comfortable that financial oversight was continuously in place. After Doctor Elkins moved to LSU as chair, he subsequently moved to Hopkins as chief of gynecology, completing a geographic and institutional flip-flop between the two of us that confused many. Unfortunately, Doctor Elkins died prematurely from an acute myocardial infarction while playing basketball with his sons. Several Ghanaian postgraduates doing rotations in the US joined me in Baltimore for his funeral, representing the GPTP that he was instrumental in establishing.

Doctor Danso became head of department at KNUST School of Medical Sciences (SMS) and at KATH upon Professor J. O. Martey's move to KNUST as vice-provost. When Danso became dean of the medical school, another GPTP graduate, Doctor Opare-Addo, became head of department (HOD) at KNUST and KATH. The pipeline was flowing.

Professor (by now) Kwawukume was soon HOD at KBTH, then K. K. Bentsi-Enchill Chair (the first endowed chair at the UGMS named after an earlier well-respected OBGYN HOD and funded by his family), and was the second Ghanaian and GPTP graduate to become an honorary fellow of ACOG. Professor Danso, who had earlier risen to the position of dean of medicine in Kumasi, was the first. As Professor Kwawukume moved up to other more senior administrative roles, Professor Samuel Obed became HOD, eventually reaching CEO of KBTH. Doctor Kwawukume, with his wife Doctor Susu Kwawukume, a dermatologist, went on to establish the first private medical school in Ghana in 2013, where he is president. The Family Health University College (FHUC) Medical School has since graduated their first class on the grounds of the Family Health Hospital where it is based (https://fhu.edu.gh), a beautiful campus directly on the Atlantic Ocean across the highway from the Kofi Annan International Peacekeeping Training Centre. I was honored when the FHUC named their library after me. The basketball court at FHMS on the FHUC grounds and overlooking the Atlantic Ocean was supported by UM alumni who visited during a trip to Ghana to travel the geographic route of the story of the GPTP. American supporters have also provided medical school scholarships and financial support for other priorities associated with the ongoing medical education and training priorities at institutions associated with the GPTP and its successors.

Doctor Richard Adanu was recognized early on as a star (much more about Doctor Adanu in Chapter 7). During his rotation at the University of Michigan, he told me he wanted to pursue an MPH. Professor Ampofo's MPH from Hopkins was a storied part of KBTH history. I lobbied old Hopkins friends, Professors Bernie Guyer and Amy Tsui from the Department of Maternal and Child Health to assist in finding funding for Adanu, which they did. Professor Bernie Guyer was chair of the Department of Maternal and Child Health at Hopkins. I had served on the search committee that identified him, and I knew he cared about the Ghana program; his wife, Jane Guyer, was a renowned Africa-focused anthropologist. As a medical student at Rochester, Guyer had done a community health elective in Nigeria, where he was inspired by a young Doctor Adetokunbo Lucas to pursue a career in public health and pediatrics. He was so inspired by Lucas that Bernie's son's middle name is Adetokunbo. More "small world" in operation. Richard Adanu got funding as a Gates scholar and did brilliantly at Hopkins, working with Professors Guyer and Tsui in maternal and child health (MCH). Adanu graduated with distinction and was elected to Delta Omega, the public health honorary. He returned to Ghana and rose meteorically from an initial faculty position in Obstetrics and Gynecology to the Department of Maternal and Child Health in the School of Public Health (SPH), and then to the Deanship of the SPH at the University of Ghana at age forty-three. The new paradigm of young leaders was established. GPTP graduates had demonstrably moved quickly through the academic pipeline to major leadership positions.

Lessons Learned

Develop a shared vision with all participants.

Local management and control!

Local leadership and local decision making!

Community-based participation works for academic programs, education, and research.

Difficult conversations are hard. They are necessary and a learned skill.

CHAPTER 5

The Continuation of the "Program" and Years Five to Twenty

It should be clear that the initial startup of the program was hard, and the first several years were challenging. There were many naysayers, roadblocks, and bumps in the road. The goodwill and desire of all concerned to achieve success moved the program forward. It also became clear to me that Lawson was a good person to have on the team because every time we went to Ghana, he sent me and others to work with the postgraduates on research and academic scholarship (publications were a focus), to teach, and to make rounds, which is what I did best. He met with the Ministry of Health. I was never interested in meeting with the MOH, and because I was naïve politically, I did not realize until later how important engagement with the MOH was. As I came from a culture of mostly autonomous academic research universities, Lawson clearly knew from experience in Africa and similar experiences in the United Kingdom that the MOH and the Ghana Health Service controlled the resources of the teaching hospital. Since the Ghana Health Service, part of the MOH, supported junior faculty and consultants after they finished residency, it was a critically important partner for the teaching hospitals in Ghana. Doctor Ken Sagoe, who represented

45

the MOH for a time on the GPTP leadership team as deputy director of the Ghana Health Service, was a brilliant colleague. He went on to be the chief executive officer of the Tamale Teaching Hospital associated with the University for Development Sciences in Tamale (Northern Region), which developed the third medical school in Ghana. In that capacity he took a very resource-limited quality institution and made it great both in terms of facility infrastructure and as a clinically and academically respectable teaching hospital. When he left, the Tamale Teaching Hospital had medical students who were getting excellent clinical rotations, and it has become a respected teaching hospital for housemen, postgraduates, and now OBGYN residents. Doctor Sagoe went on to become a special counselor for health to the president of Ghana (and his daughter, as a medical student at KNUST, was selected by her dean for a Michigan senior student rotation, see Chapter 6).

Two graduates of the GPTP, Doctor Gumanga from KBTH in Accra and Doctor David Kolbilla, a KATH trainee who was among the very first cohort of family planning and reproductive health fellowship graduates from Kumasi, went to Tamale to become the first full-time fully trained obstetrics and gynecology consultants at the Tamale Teaching Hospital. Before that, visiting Cuban doctors had provided services at Tamale. Shortly thereafter, they started getting four-year OBGYN trainee graduates from the new four-year Ghana College of Physicians and Surgeons (GCPS) "membership" training program. With this influx of well-trained specialists, high-quality clinical service became available in the enhanced Tamale Teaching Hospital that Doctor Sagoe had made possible. Maternity and maternal outcomes improved, and given Kolbilla's training and experience, enhanced safe abortion services were provided in the clinics and hospital as well. It did not take long for Kolbilla to be recognized for his administrative skills in medical care service and as HOD, and soon after Doctor Ken Sagoe left Tamale, Kolbilla became CEO of the Tamale Teaching Hospital.

It was very important that the Ghana Health Service (the physician services branch of the MOH that employed and posted physicians) and the MOH be involved in the program. The mix of Americans and Europeans on the External Advisory Board really benefited the program planning. It was clear that the American system encouraged people to be successful. The Americans felt that if people failed, it was the teacher's or the system's fault, in contrast to the archaic and slowly fading European model, where it was the student's own fault for failure, and where sometimes "how many students you could fail" reflected positively on the professor. Multiple-choice questions (MCQs) became standard for examinations rather than open-ended essay questions, which had been the standard and were invariably graded arbitrarily and not objectively. Oral examinations were often given by some American participants so that American techniques used from American Board of Obstetrics and Gynecologists (ABOG) examinations were clearly articulated. Ghanaian faculty eventually traveled to the ABOG testing center in Dallas to personally observe American exams in preparation and in process. The consistent and careful attention to test questions and test metrics, often based on material in the Ghanaian texts as the sources (see below), facilitated early on the remarkable successes of Ghanaian trainees. The pass rate for Ghanaians soon after the program started, both on Part 1 and Part 2, rapidly became very high (over 90 percent), especially compared to the Nigerian pass rate (40 percent). In addition, the publication of the first local textbook *Comprehensive Obstetrics in the Tropics* in 2002 (Kwawukume & Emuveyan, 2002), edited by E.Y. Kwawukume and well-known Nigerian professor E. Ejiro Emuveyan, and written entirely by West Africans, mostly Ghanaians, provided a textbook that was reliable and easy to read. This text provided another clinical guidebook for residents and students to follow that allowed them to achieve very high scores on their examinations. This book and subsequent published texts were paperback and available for about thirty dollars, much less expensive than the several-hundred-dollar hardcover texts available before then. The text was an immediate success, and it became even more successful when it was reviewed very positively in the prestigious British journal, the *Lancet*, of Rosenfield "Where is the M in MCH?" fame:

> At first glance, I was somewhat skeptical about how *Comprehensive Obstetrics in the Tropics* could possibly improve on the standard set by the classic text *Obstetrics and Gynaecology in the Tropics and Developing Countries*, first published in 1967 by John Lawson and David Stewart,

and the recently updated version, *Maternity Care in Developing Countries*, by John Lawson, Kelsey Harrison, and Staffan Bergström. But I was pleased to find another valuable and useful reference for students and medical educators of women's health in less-developed countries. Given the expanding body of rigorously appraised published work on effectiveness of obstetric care, the arrival of this textbook is timely. In addition, books such as this one that are published regionally are a readily accessible source of valuable information for health professionals who work in Africa. The textbook is informative and easy to read. Important aspects of preconception and prenatal care, HIV infection in pregnancy, and practical aspects of obstetric procedures are discussed. Other topics that are reviewed include high maternal mortality in the tropics and predisposing factors, such as unsafe abortion, obstructed labour, and obstetric haemorrhage.

(Olatunbosun 2002)

With this review of a locally edited, written, and published obstetric textbook in the *Lancet*, many GPTP graduates, especially the academics, felt the program had truly achieved world-class status; it had certainly achieved world-class recognition. It was a signal benchmark in the development of the GPTP.

The first textbook was soon followed by *Comprehensive Gynaecology in the Tropics* (2005), which soon supplanted the long-outdated and out-of-print, but still commonly used and referenced, 1967 text *Obstetrics and Gynaecology in the Tropics and Developing Countries* by John Lawson. Professor Lawson often talked about and long aspired to update his book, but a couple of attempts never achieved the popularity or renown of the original (Lawson & Harrison, 1995; Lawson et al., 2001). Lawson died before seeing this important achievement of the Ghanaian textbooks. He would have been pleased—and would have found it entirely appropriate—that definitive new texts were written entirely by West African authors from Ghana and his beloved Nigeria. The Ghana medical students soon did extremely well with very high pass rates in obstetrics and gynecology. The success rates on the medical student examinations both in Accra and Kumasi were the highest in obstetrics and gynecology because the students were given these books to study, they knew what they needed to learn, and they were tested on that material. This was very emblematic of the American educational system, where you tell people what they need to know, give them the relevant and appropriate material to achieve competency, and then test them on what they have learned.

Thus, in the early years, a recognizable GPTP model emerged, and subsequently many other training programs in Ghana have followed its design. The GPTP was first described in a peer-reviewed publication by Professor Cecil Klufio, who had returned to Ghana from Papua New Guinea and assumed the position as director of the GPTP in Accra. It appeared in the prominent "high-impact" *American Journal of Obstetrics and Gynecology* (Klufio et al., 2003), and the subsequent successes and retention of the trainees were described in papers by Doctor Frank Anderson and other colleagues (Anderson et al., 2007; Clinton, 2010). These papers used survey methodologies to determine why postgraduates stayed in Ghana as opposed to seeking further opportunities abroad, especially in high-income countries in the Global North. The presence of a high-quality in-country training program was crucial. It was clear that Ghana's recognition of quality and pride in the programs was an early and important effect. Economic and political stability were also important. Finally, the early and subsequent data show that the themes of being able to give back to their country, love for the nation, and caring for their own communities in close proximity to their own nuclear and extended families were consistently expressed by the program graduates.

Subsequent attempts to identify detailed perceived reasons for the successes of the program revealed long-term partnership, local management, transparency, capacity building, sustainability, and personal relationships as the major factors identified. It is interesting that we will see very similar factors reappear when we describe the Charter process (Chapter 8) that attempts to carefully define the optimal approaches to collaboration between high-income and low-income academic institutions around health care capacity building.

Lessons Learned—Ghana: Why They Stayed and Why It Worked

- IN-COUNTRY TRAINING
- POLITICAL AND ECONOMIC STABILITY
- NATIONAL AND SOCIAL TIES
- LONG-TERM PARTNERSHIP
- LOCAL MANAGEMENT AND CONTROL
- BILATERAL EXCHANGE
- TRANSPARENCY (FINANCIAL, ADMINISTRATION, ETC.)
- CAPACITY BUILDING
- LONG-TERM SUSTAINABILITY
- PERSONAL RELATIONSHIPS AND COMMITMENT

(from Anderson et al., 2007; Clinton et al., 2010)

It was very important that the program and its progress and evaluations be described academically through peer-reviewed publications. What was described could then serve as a pathway and guide for future programs. One of the intentional paths that we took throughout the development and maturation of the program was to make sure we reported on it regularly. It was the first paper that was presented orally before a large audience in 2002 by Professor Cecil Klufio at APGO that got many Americans interested in the potential for opportunities in global health. In retrospect, the fact that we published regularly and published a careful description of the developing program for others to follow and replicate as appropriate became important when it came to replication projects. Reading these publications would lead people looking for successful models of locally developed postgraduate medical training to the Ghana model (Chapter 10). Many of these papers were part of the individual academic advancement of the Ghanaians and formed the basis of my own developing reputation in global health. As has become clear from the beginning, the GPTP was embedded in the universities. I was an academic. I understood the academy. My life had been focused on developing the careers of people in the academy. Teaching medical students, encouraging those interested to go into obstetrics and gynecology, supporting them throughout their careers (one of my students, Andy Satin, had support from me in his residency application, did a maternal-fetal medicine fellowship, returned to chair the department at his alma mater USUHS, and now has been director at Johns Hopkins for over a decade, and we have moved from mentor/mentees to colleagues and friends).

By 2014, global health was all the rage (Erikson & Wendland, 2014; Kidder, 2003; Stagg et al., 2017) and, in my opinion, too many students were following a less than rigorous and sustainable approach to global health. At the University of Michigan, we had medical students in the same class who had started NGOs in the same country as undergraduates with no knowledge of their competition or similarities. Most of these NGOs will not have the sustained effect that university-based programs can have if they do commit their institution priorities (which include sustainability and survival) with their global initiatives and global partners. The Charter project distilled these principles (see Chapter 7). The Gates Charter project and Charter for Collaboration provided the opportunity to memorialize, record, and publish the principles that had evolved and developed with the GPTP. We were able to bring together the various stakeholders—UGMS, KNUST, MOH—at the resort next to the historical Elmina Castle near Cape Coast to talk about shared vision and shared values. This weeklong meeting bringing interdisciplinary in-country stakeholders together often allowed them to share discussion in a non-rushed fashion and sometimes meet face-to-face for the first time. Michigan and Frank W. J. Anderson served as conveners; the University of Michigan, as a public institution that values and models interdisciplinarity, had become a trusted and valuable partner.

In Ghana at the time, private universities were a rarity, so for most people universities were public institutions serving the public good. This aligned well with University of Michigan's own goals as a public institution, and one consistently committed in word and deed to serving the public good. And the University of Michigan owned its own hospital and a large academic medical center. Ghanaian universities were similar. University leaders in Ghana, often unaware of this difference between public and private institutions in the global context (remember, Ghana was heavily influenced by the United Kingdom, where many if not most of the oldest and most distinguished universities are public, not private, unlike the United States) had not previously appreciated this significant difference among well-known American universities. Understanding the common public mission, they were able to identify and relate to the similarities between the University of Michigan and major Ghanaian universities in their public nature and see a Michigan-Ghana partnership as an advantage. The major difference was that in Ghana there were the government ministries (MOH for the medical schools and health-related programs, Ministry of Education, or MOE, for the universities, and sometimes, to make things complicated, both the MOH and MOE could be involved in academic medical financing, programs, and policies). There is no clear US equivalent in most cases, and this difference mandated that in Ghana the MOH needed to be at the table from the very start of discussions about academic collaboration, an early and critical lesson from John Lawson. American university participants (including me, early on) were more used to a model where universities had much more autonomy and certainly not the same degree of dependency and control from an outside government entity. Understanding cultural differences sometimes took time and repeated collaborative discussions.

When the program was started in 1989, the West African College of Physicians and Surgeons (often just WACS, since that was the college's home of obstetrics and gynecology engagement, the WACP being for internists and non-surgeons) was the only accrediting and professional body for medical specialties, so a five-year program was developed to meet the established WACS requirements for fellowship. This program ultimately would lead to a large number of trained, boarded specialists who have since populated the academic ranks and gone on to many other positions in the ranks of professional service and practice. It remains arguably the most desirable and prestigious qualification for those people receiving training in Ghana. Eventually there were so many Ghanaian trainees taking the WACS exams that a second testing site (previously all WACS exams were given in Ibadan) was established for the Part 1 and the Part 2 examinations in Accra. From the very beginning, the GPTP faculty and participants recognized that in Nigeria there was also a Nigerian College of Obstetrics and Gynecology that had separate board examinations, and many Nigerians were fellows of both the West African College of Surgeons and the Nigerian College.

Ghanaians soon had a desire to develop their own college, and eventually the Ghana College of Physicians and Surgeons was established as the "National Postgraduate Medical College established to train specialist doctors in medicine, surgery and other related disciplines" by an Act of Parliament in 2003. The Ghana College of Physicians and Surgeons sought to train specialists and subspecialists in Ghana for Ghanaian practice. The Ghana College had a different model from the West African College of Surgeons. Ghana used a British-derived model that included training for membership (member of the Ghana College of Surgeons, MGCS,) which only required four years of training, with the idea that two or three years of further practice with some evidence of scholarship and teaching would lead to fellowship. (This leads to some confusion, as subspecialty trainees are usually designated as fellows or fellows in training, while "fellowship" is often used to describe those who have been accepted into professional societies in the United States, e.g., Fellow of the American College of Obstetricians and Gynecologists or Fellow of the American College of Surgeons, or in the United Kingdom, Fellow of Royal Colleges. Some professional societies like the Royal Colleges and the American College of Physicians have a lower "membership level," which does not exist in ACOG or ACS.) Another road to fellowship in the Ghanaian College of Surgeons would be subspecialty (fellowship) training such as family planning and reproductive health, urogynecology, maternal-fetal medicine, oncology, etc. These fellowships have been developed (Dalton et al., 2013). The presence of these two college options has led to some people to pursue both credentials, requiring them to register and pay dues to both the West African College of Surgeons and the Ghana College of Physicians and Surgeons. Here again, gamesmanship and medical politics came into play. Many of the Ghanaians now complete their Ghana College "membership" and are practicing throughout the country side-by-side with people who have trained for five years in programs of the West African College of Surgeons. The doctors from the early days were grandfathered into the Ghanaian society when it was established, so they were fellows of both the West African College of Surgeons and the Ghana College of Physicians and Surgeons in the faculty of obstetrics and gynecology. Those who do not want to pursue short and long commentaries (detailed clinical essays) and undergo the trials of the West African College of Surgeons oral examinations finish with a "membership" in the GCPS, become MGCS, and practice as obstetrician/gynecologists throughout the country. They may not have as much surgical training as the five-year FWACS, but they are able to handle the majority of medical issues and routine surgeries very well.

Most people who are interested in academics now either pursue the West African College of Surgeons or register early for further obstetric/gynecologic subspecialization in gynecologic oncology, family planning, urogynecology or maternal-fetal medicine and through their subspecialization and dissertation receive fellowship in the Ghana College of Surgeons (FGCS).

The first subspecialization to be launched in Ghana was the reproductive health and family planning (RHFP) fellowship training program, thanks to funding from an anonymous foundation. These initial fellows, who completed the training in 2011, have been very successful in introducing family planning and contraception countrywide. Complex family planning was a late-developing fellowship in the United States, yet it was the first fellowship to be accepted in Ghana, since family planning, contraceptive uptake, and safe abortion were a national public health and medical priority and because foundation funding was available. The first four fellows went on to successful activities in both program development and management in family planning, with several going on to become heads of department (e.g., Doctor David Kolbilla in Tamale and Doctor Emmanuel Morhe in Ho). After four years of anonymous external foundation funding of the RHFP fellowship, like the GPTP, ongoing financial support for RHFP fellowship training was assumed by the MOH (Dalton et al., 2013).

Unfortunately, some people were caught in a "donut hole," having begun their training when the West African College of Surgeons existed, but not the Ghana College, and then finished after the Ghana College had come into being, but were not considered senior enough to be grandfathered into fellowship. When they went on to take their fellowship entry examinations, they were not approved to sit for the exams since they had not registered with the Ghana College when they started, nor were they members of the Ghana College. These few people caught in the donut hole represented another administrative and political challenge illustrating that political issues, administrative issues, and transnational issues, such as competition between the West African College of Surgeons and the Ghana College of Physicians and Surgeons, provide similar challenges in Africa as they often can in the United States. This was very frustrating for me. I felt very bad for those few excellent people in the donut hole. I wrote letters, I sent emails, but with no effect. Eventually, with time, those who had been left out found a way to accomplish their academic goals, the donut hole closed, and all were satisfied with the outcome. People talk about "Africa time." It is clearly different from the American mindset to resolve any possible issues or human resources problem expeditiously. Like with our push to get certain faculty promoted in the early years of the GPTP, the Ghanaians were best left to manage their own administrative, bureaucratic, and sometimes cultural and idiosyncratic issues themselves and in their own time.

Lessons Learned

Support and develop academic leaders.
Don't forget the Ministry of Health!
Respect local institutions and institutional process.
Political and economic stability is a key factor in people's hope for
their country's future and their own.

CHAPTER 6

Students and Other Learners

From the early days of the postgraduate training program, resident exchanges were part of the program (Klufio et al., 2003; Anderson et al., 2007). Ghana senior residents came to the United States for two to three months to finish off their case books, a requirement for Part 2 of the WACS exams, with the goal of having them complete their short commentaries (three- to five-page case summaries), their long commentaries (thirty- to forty-page discussions of a clinical problem or often, resident-performed research), and have practice sessions with US faculty to be prepared for their oral examinations. In addition, they were being introduced to technology unavailable in Ghana, such as electronic fetal monitoring, endoscopic surgery, and advanced imaging techniques. In the early years, the priority was on providing the opportunity to graduating senior residents, since we really did not want junior residents to be seduced by the technology or seduced into the idea that they could complete their training in high-income countries and remain. This turned out to be very successful, as this preparation before examinations led to a pass rate of nearly 100 percent, and often learners were able to develop quite a critical insight on the overuse of technology in the United States, where patients received ultrasounds, MRIs, CTs (advanced imaging techniques), and all sorts of laboratory tests. The Ghanaians were able to see that while they lacked much of the advanced technology, we Americans used technology in a way that produced its own problems (overuse, delay in diagnosis, high cost, waste of resources). These technologies, including ultrasound, electronic fetal monitoring, and CT scans, have subsequently been introduced in Ghana, where they have been used more sparingly and, arguably, more rationally as well.

Since the resident exchanges from Ghana to the United States were successful, shortly after I moved to Michigan, we encouraged residents from Michigan to go to Ghana for rotations in their third and fourth year. Luckily, we had an elective rotation where residents could do this, and the expanded exchange program turned out to be quite successful. Every year, one or two residents would go and come back with new perspectives, and it was transformational for some, such as Doctor Senait Fisseha who, as we shall see later (Chapter 10), recognized the successes and opportunities in Ghana to inform those that she was subsequently able to achieve in Ethiopia.

Once we had successful resident exchanges established, it was clear that the exchange of medical students was something we should consider next. From the beginning of the medical student exchange program, the intentional principle was that at least an equal number of students should come to Michigan from Ghana as went from Michigan to Ghana, and we aimed for a 2:1 ratio, Ghana to Michigan. This fundamental equity was an essential and consistent part of the department's global health ethos (Chapter 8). Funding was a challenge, but we were able from the very beginning to make this bilateral exchange part of our department priorities, and eventually part of the department mission and strategy. It was an excellent way to recruit the best students and residents interested in global health to Ann Arbor from all over the United States. The US medical students went to Ghana, usually either Accra or Kumasi (Lawrence et al., 2020), and eventually to Ethiopia, and stayed in student housing, often international student housing with medical students from all over the world.

These opportunities provided remarkable clinical experience for these fourth-year medical students. One of the differences between medical students and physician exchanges is the difference in professional status. Any postgraduate medical trainee from Ghana or the United States who is part of the clinical exchange is required to get a medical license. It has been relatively easy for US doctors to get short-term temporary licenses in Ghana, although this is slowly evolving to be more costly as the Ghana Medical and Dental Council (GMDC) sees an opportunity to increase its fees and foreign exchange. It is generally prohibitively expensive and time-consuming for Ghanaians to get even temporary US licenses. This has been one inequity that has been difficult to overcome (Hudspeth et al., 2019), but the Ghana physicians already have substantial clinical hands-on experience, so they have been satisfied to attend teaching conferences, clinical rounds, and observe clinical care. Everything but touching a patient and providing medical advice and services is permitted. For those Ghanaians needing surgical training or hands-on experience, such as gynecologic oncology fellows, meaningful experiences have been arranged in South Africa, Singapore, Cambodia, and other sites where temporary licenses and high volumes of cases make quality clinical experiences possible. Medical students have been accepted on both sides of the Ghana partnership as learners in training and are able to participate meaningfully in clinical care under faculty supervision. Issues of malpractice coverage have been covered by mutually acceptable memoranda of understanding. Visiting senior medical students from Michigan and Ghana have been able to participate in deliveries, scrub on (participate in) operations, and truly see what professional medical life is like in a comparatively very different environment and country. The Michigan students received excellent teaching from faculty members whom we had had the privilege to train as residents and who were part of high-quality educational training programs with local medical students who were equally well read and highly competent. One of the major things our medical students learned was the high quality of the practice of medicine they saw, despite the lack of resources and lack of equipment available in their home country. They were also able to see such diseases as malaria and see labor progressing and managed in ways that were eye-opening. This was a challenge sometimes. My son, as a fourth-year medical student, traveled to Accra, where he was a member of the team whose faculty members I knew and had trained. He was galvanized to be able to scrub in cesarean section rooms where the electric lights went out and operations were done by candlelight, but he was taken aback to see a multiparous woman die from postpartum hemorrhage and lack of blood, and another woman with a septic abortion managed by a traditional healer die in the emergency room. To some extent, I think this early introduction to maternal mortality might have been too much that early in his career, and we will see if he follows my path in global initiatives as he has followed my path as an obstetrician and a maternal-fetal medicine specialist.

The students from Ghana came to the University of Michigan on a regular basis, and initially we took students just from Accra and Kumasi, but as new medical schools were established and medical students matured to senior-year clinical rotations in Tamale and Cape Coast, we had to reduce the number of students from each site, given the increasing numbers of Ghana medical students. The program became quite competitive, and we have left it to the dean's office at each of the Ghana medical schools to develop a process to select those students who are offered rotations at Michigan. We provided them with housing and a small stipend, but they had to provide their own travel money. This led to a certain uncomfortable elitism, since only the students who had the resources to travel came to the United States for these one-month rotations as senior medical students. Income disparity, often geographically determined by living in large urban areas, is a major challenge in Ghanaian culture and society. Their rotations to Michigan were almost always excellent, with the Ghana students not only impressing the University of Michigan students and faculty with their knowledge but also being able to see doctor-patient relationships and the high degree to which patients were educated in patient-centered practices by physicians in the United States. The commitment to shared decision making, patient autonomy, and the detailed process of informed consent was noted by many (Abedini et al., 2014, 2015; Danso-Bamfo et al., 2017). They were able to see the individual patient rooms in the Labor and Delivery area, quite different from delivery spaces in Ghana, and in joining residents, faculty, and nurse midwives they saw different approaches to interprofessional care that many were determined to take back with them for their practice. The students repeatedly articulated the fact that they were energized by how much information they had gained, but also felt confident after coming to the United States that they had already received a world-class education in Ghana. What stuck with them was the differences in the physician-patient relationship in a patient-centered environment, the more humanistic way patients were cared for by the nurses, and the potential use and overuse of technology as well. The electronic medical record was an important aspect of their learning.

The American students going to Ghana learned a different set of priorities and skills. The Americans were humbled by the high quality of the faculty, trainees, and medical students they met in Ghana and gained a new understanding of tropical diseases and conditions. The Ghanaians came to recognize the world-class quality of the medical education they were receiving in their home country despite high levels of maternal mortality and a lack of technological resources. Both groups of students returned home with a better understanding of health services, health systems, and global challenges to health. Since understanding health systems is part of the developing, internationally recognized implicit curriculum, this was no doubt useful as part of their education. The Ghanaian students learned about humanism, engagement, patient education, patient interactions, informed consent, the concept of patient-centered care, the relatively high level of medical literacy of many patients in the United States, and the clinical use (and overuse) of technology. They are asked to write their personal reflections, and it is always gratifying to see the strong self-reflective and self-aware responses they have had (Abedini et al., 2015; Danso-Bamfo et al., 2017).

I have followed many of these students on a shared Facebook site and have kept track of their careers. A very few outstanding students have followed up on their lifelong desire to come to the United States, but the vast majority have completed training in Ghana, many in obstetrics and gynecology. We have had spouses of former exchange medical students come from Ghana as residents and fellows, and there are ongoing interactions between the Ghanaian and Michigan students at all levels on their own Facebook page called "Maize, blue, red, gold, green lounge," referencing the Ghanaian national colors of red, gold, and green and the maize and blue of Michigan.

In addition to clinical activities, the Ghana students often attended football games, where they loved the Michigan "Big House" and the marching band; basketball games, where they loved the cheerleaders and smaller, but energetic, pep band; social events like Fourth of July picnics; visits to African World Festival celebrations and the Charles H. Wright Museum of African American History in Detroit; kayaking or canoeing down the Huron River; and often for many, Sunday church.

The students' education also fostered a very rich and often long-lasting relationship with key Michigan administrative staff, especially Jennifer Jones in the OBGYN department, who organized many of their clinical rotations and kept calendars of teaching activities up to date, and Carrie Ashton from Global REACH, who arranged housing and weekend events and even hosted parties that got her special recognition with the honorific "Mama Duck." Because there were so many questions about travel, immunizations, clothing, etc., early on we developed a very detailed and useful handbook for travel that is revised and updated regularly by all those who travel to Ghana and come back. This is a great institutional resource for all global program travelers and is a best practice that should be developed locally by any institution developing global partnerships (Appendix 3).

On the Ghana side, Mercy and Patience are two of the long-time secretaries in the Department of Obstetrics and Gynecology at the University of Ghana who were invaluable in helping me during my early trips to Ghana. Not only were they able to facilitate finding student housing for visiting Michigan students and residents, but they also arranged weekend trips for them to Kakum National Park, with its walkway over the tropical rain forest, the moving Elmina Castle, and the Mole National Park, with its animal reserve northwest of Tamale in the Northern Region. Patience and Mercy had excellent connections to low-cost excursion and tour companies and contacts for almost anything else the students needed or wanted. All of this led to a closeness and often to sustained online relationships among all students, staff, and residents on both sides of the Ghana partnership who recognized and appreciated the special importance of these shared experiences and personal relationships.

I think one of the real benefits of having the medical exchange program has been the stability of the Ghana administrative staff and reliable housing available to accept students in the same international guest houses in Accra and Kumasi. Arranging for comfortable and accessible housing for Ghanaian students in the United States for close and convenient access to public transportation so they can get to morning report and rounds really adds to their experience. Bus service in Ann Arbor is not as reliable for transportation as it is in Ghana. In addition to the academic support issues, having reliable and consistent administrative personnel on the ground is also important for rapid changes or requests, often so that we can say to any student who is selected by their medical school and makes last-minute arrangements that we can accommodate changes in our clinical rotation quickly. All this administrative infrastructure and capacity represents what we have come to call our Global REACH "platform." Countries and sites where we have long-standing academic partnerships and established administrative capacity to support a substantial number of Michigan students, projects, and programs, often across the university. We have also, not infrequently, facilitated requests from students from outside the University of Michigan to participate in clinical opportunities in Ghana.

In addition to the resident exchanges and medical student exchanges, we now have fellowship exchanges. Fellows from Ghana have come to do advanced gynecologic oncology in conjunction with Doctor Carolyn Johnston, and Doctor Gabriel Ganyaglo did an extended period of study in urogynecology with Doctor John Delancey. In this way, they have truly experienced a world-class finishing school and preparation to be outstanding practicing subspecialists. The same type of resident exchange has now happened with maternal-fetal medicine faculty and fellows from Ghana and from St. Paul's Hospital Millennium Medical College in Ethiopia (Chapter 10). Again, the bilaterality of the exchanges among faculty, fellows, residents, and medical students is an important component of this collaboration. It is most easily achieved in the context of long-term sustained collaborations between institutions that can accommodate the learners both pedagogically and administratively, and with respect to housing, food, and a little fun on the side. The totality of the experience is an important part of a successful partnership. These repetitive exchanges, the organizational and administrative ability to do this consistently and well, vast institutional access to clinical faculty and educational resources, and institutional memory are all an important part of this process. At Michigan, the Global REACH office, the medical school's global health hub (https://medicine.umich.edu/dept/globalreach), is the central organizational point of contact and critical in all it has done to help with the myriad demands and requirements of international exchanges and global health engagement programs.

When he became dean of the medical school, Doctor James Woolliscroft, who was a respected medical educator himself, established for the first time at Michigan an intentional global health program for medical students, based in Global REACH. One of his excellent, in my mind, initiatives was to make up to $1,000 available to any senior (fourth-year) UM medical student to pursue an international training opportunity. Doctor David Stern was an excellent initial choice as the inaugural director of Global REACH, and his speaker series, scholarship distribution to first- and second-year medical students ("M1s and M2s"), and other initiatives for global research proposals and programmatic initiatives were successful in making more and more students aware of global offerings and supporting those students who were already seeking them. Doctor Stern was recruited to Mount Sinai in New York. I was asked to assume the directorship of Global REACH. At the time, a new senior executive associate dean for education and global initiatives, Doctor Joseph Kolars, had been recruited from the Mayo Clinic and was expected to arrive within a year. I thought the direction and leadership of Global REACH should be decided by Doctor Kolars, so I accepted an <u>interim</u> position directing Global REACH with the agreement that I would cede the permanent position to Doctor Kolars upon his arrival. I continued Doctor Stern's programs and attended as many of the student sessions as I could. One of the major student projects entirely conceived and managed by the student Global REACH chapter was what they called "service mission trips." These trips were mostly to Central and South America by M1s, since the schedules of M2s and M3s were essentially a full twelve months.

This leads to the need to introduce a topology of the major types of medical student engagement in global health:

A Topology of Global Health Engagement

- Missionary work—service, sometimes proselytization
- Service-learning trips (paid organizers)
- Medical tourism (medical voyeurism)—paid or unpaid organizers (sometimes involves minimal service)
- Medical student "white coat" programs
- "Professional" exchanges—high-level, high-tech, travel-involved (e.g., oncology, cardiology, or neurosurgery centers) usually paid for by participants, often led by senior physicians (substantial gender disparities among medical professionals, male dominance, paternalism, elite)
- Surgical programs (Operation Smile, Project HOPE, Global Sight Alliance)
- NGOs—JHIEPGO, MSI Reproductive Choices, John Snow, Engender Health
- University-based, pedagogically and developmentally appropriate curricular offerings for medical students and health science advanced learners

One can see the various options, starting with the types of service-learning trips we are describing, which can be organized by religious entities as missionary trips or by first-year medical students as service-learning trips. Organized, fee-paid service-learning trips can be fairly superficial with significant structure and minimal true experiential contact, closely approaching medical voyeurism (Anderson & Wansom, 2009; Crump & Sugarman, 2008), with an "Oh my gosh, can you believe people live like this? You would not believe the hospital facilities!" type of reaction and response. Occasionally such experiences do instill a lifelong commitment to global health equity that can be achieved by more intentional and structured global health experiences, but often the visitors never return or make another service trip again.

The professional exchanges described are often high-cost experiences for doctors from high-income countries to visit institutions of high quality, often cancer institutes, heart centers, or other high-technology, super-specialized care. In many parts of the world, these centers are led by medical elites, often men in surgical or high-acuity specialties. The long-term impact and sustainable effects and outcomes of these trips are unclear to me.

Surgical programs, such as Operation Smile and similar programs, that "repair" often complex childhood conditions where there is no local capacity certainly can have long-term benefits for those lucky enough to receive their service. They have been criticized for their lack of postoperative care and follow-up, which are often necessary for such conditions as vesicovaginal fistula, cleft lip repair, and neurosurgical repairs, where the surgical failure rate can be quite high. Good examples of consistently successful surgical programs are ophthalmologic interventions for cataracts and simple eye surgeries that can be vision sparing and sight improving and can be done quickly and safely with minimal surgical failures or postoperative services. (Heisel et al., 2020, 2021).

NGOs have excellent global health programs and are highly present in this space. The major critique is that they often depend on grant funding and foundation support, and their programs are therefore often financially at risk of three or five-year funding cycles. They also are dependent on the financial priorities of the funders and can risk not being intentional or focused in their programmatic planning. Function—the activities of the NGO and their direction—depends on funding.

As you can imagine, I am a proponent of academic partnerships for many of the reasons that I have already mentioned. Sustainability is one of the major ones: I often say that universities are the second-greatest and longest-standing institution of Western civilization after the Church.

Now, back to the issue of student service mission trips, which appear as "medical student 'white coat' programs," and a few other programs in the above rubric. (White coats signify clinical engagement with patients and really are most appropriately donned by students as they begin their patient engagements. They became the "official dress" of doctors at the turn of the twentieth century, when laboratory science became more important in medical practice with the microscope and other laboratory devices being associated with clean, white lab coats. Recently, medical schools have mounted "white coat ceremonies" for medical students and their family to recognize their achievement in being accepted to medical school, often preceding even the first day of class without much other introduction to the profession. Personally, I do not wear a white coat because of the power structure it suggests. I find white coat ceremonies concerning; rather than being lauded by their families and future professors, I think the most important issues to inculcate in new students are those of humility and acceptance of the challenges associated with being a physician. Professional power should not even be suggested this early in professional development.) When I was interim director of Global REACH, I became concerned when I learned the M1s were receiving instruction from M2s on patient care and interactions—not the full curricular faculty directed and taught Introduction to the Patient course required of all M2s, but rather a fast introduction to clinical skills, including history taking, blood pressure measurement, cardiac auscultations, and other seemingly simple "doctor skills" for use during upcoming "service-learning" trips.

This was concerning to me. I felt students should learn clinical skills from faculty in a full curriculum that included a broad introduction to history taking, doctor-patient communication skills, detailed education about the physical examination, and other parts of what is now a "doctoring curriculum," including breaking bad news, doctor-patient confidentiality, and informed consent. After discussion with students in several settings, Global REACH stopped supporting this premature "doctoring" training. I felt white coats were <u>earned</u> after the medical curriculum encompassing basic science, clinical skills, and doctoring had been introduced academically, professionally, and socially to students and when they began their clinical clerkships and were permitted to interact with patients as doctors-to-be in the hospital and clinics. The first principle, for me, was that students are developmentally and professionally not prepared to begin clinical interactions until they have received this professional education and training. Permitting this "white coat tourism" and "white coat voyeurism," I felt, was not ethical or moral from professional and institutional perspectives (Anderson & Wansom, 2009). These students doing global work represented our institution when they participated in the work and needed proper training. Equally important, their premature clinical presence represented our institutional standards and priorities poorly. Even though it was student-run, it was nonetheless an affiliated program, and students going out were representing Michigan as an institution with a "block M" on their white short coat.

Secondly, as part of this thought exercise, we needed to ask whether we would let professionally unprepared international medical students come to the United States to offer similar "service." I often asked, "Would we let untrained and unprepared students from ____ (pick any South American or Central American country, or for that matter ANY foreign country) come to ____ (fill in the blank, say, inner-city Detroit or Cleveland) for service-learning trips not fully supervised, much less unprepared clinically and culturally by their home institution?" This was clearly not good medical education. It does not take into account the necessary developmental professional preparation for medical practice that occurs incrementally over the course of four years of medical school. It is disrespectful, if not unethical, in its approach to underserved, disadvantaged, low-income people and populations in need.

Any disregard of an individual's humanity and global social injustice and inequity being most important for me, Global REACH developed policies to <u>strongly</u> support supervised clinical experiences for students who had completed the clinical skills, introduction to the patient, doctoring, and clinical rotations in the various specialties (medicine, surgery, pediatrics, psychiatry, neurology, OBGYN, and emergency and family medicine being the core). This meant M4s and advanced M3 students. That said, Global REACH began emphasizing and explicitly articulating what I felt were appropriate global experiences for pre-clinical students (M1s and M2s): biomedical research, especially clinical research, and "health education" programs for underserved communities using public health and preventive primary health principles that had been introduced during class time and coursework. These students were encouraged to do health education outreach at global health centers, clinics, schools, and public venues. Experience in population health education and outreach would serve these future doctors well and give them leadership skills in advocacy and activism by seeing firsthand the needs and health aspirations of communities. In the modern age, PowerPoint slides developed and "left behind" were skills that local medical students and health care workers could continue to use after the students left. Middle and secondary school students especially love these medical student teachers—they are close in age, academically successful, and from another country. Often English was the first foreign language they had learned in school, and they wanted to practice both hearing and speaking a foreign language. These were students who could grow up to be medical students or other health science or biomedical engineering students in their own country and, eventually, successful professionals. They could become what these visiting foreign doctors-to-be were becoming.

Research, another option for the preclinical students, taught critical thinking, study design, and data collection. But more importantly, it served as a point of entry into the space of clinical encounters, clinical charts, clinical narrative, and the doctor-patient relationship. Equally important, evidence-based medicine was something all these students were going to be immersed in during their entire professional lives, and learning how evidence was collected, how studies were run, how data were analyzed, and how results were presented and published gave important insight into how evidence is generated in modern Western medicine. It is useful to know how the "sausage is made" and critical to understand how what is known and practiced today can change when new data or new practice standards are embraced. There are several types of research that medical students can pursue, and it is useful to review in a simple, descriptive way the types of disciplinary research that happens at university, first across the various university departments, then research that is predominantly biomedical:

Research across the University/Academy

HUMANITIES (primary sources): English, history

SOCIAL SCIENCE (survey, quantitative/qualitative methods): sociology, psychology, anthropology, economics, political science

BASIC SCIENCE (laboratory research, aka "bench" research): chemistry, physics, biology, biochemistry, physiology, cell and molecular biology, biomedical engineering

BIOMEDICAL RESEARCH (basic science, translational research, clinical research, outcomes research, health services, health policy, implementation science)

Biomedical Research

BASIC SCIENCE RESEARCH: molecular, animal

TRANSLATIONAL RESEARCH: "bench to bedside"

CLINICAL RESEARCH: case (clinical) studies, randomized clinical trials (RCTs)

OUTCOMES RESEARCH (outcomes of care, results of surgery or other interventions, quality, safety)

HEALTH SERVICES RESEARCH: programs, policy, case study

Research has been demonstrated to be a strong predictor of professional success in STEMM (science, technology, engineering, mathematics, and medicine), and I have always, at all levels, supported scientific research across the domains of basic, translational, clinical, health services and outcomes research, and implementation science.

In the Ghana program, we have seen that research and scholarship, including publication, have been required of residents in training and strongly supported for faculty as part of their academic career development. And for all physicians, understanding the scientific evidence basis of their practice, with lifelong attention to learning updates and keeping up with new knowledge, is key to professionalism, not to mention quality and patient safety.

The Ghana experience and Global REACH had made me very conscious of the importance of professional education and socialization that is developmentally appropriate for the stage of learning, stage of learner, and the implicit and explicit understanding of the way medical students are molded, socialized, and professionalized (and hopefully not brutalized) during the four-year US model of medical education. In a similar way, specialist residents and postgraduates are molded, professionalized, and socialized during their training, following models that were laid down in the United States by formative schools, such as the Johns Hopkins Hospital model of graduated "intern," "resident," and "fellow" training, in what has become the modern academic medical center. Under my direction, Global REACH became a very "professional development"–focused program with intentional programs that emphasized research and health education programs for preclinical medical students and clinical experiences for senior students. This professional development ontogeny is captured in the following table:

Developmentally Appropriate Ontogeny for Professionalization of Future Physicians in Medical School

- Professionalization and socialization (M1 to M4)
- Patient education/teaching (health behavior, health education), basic science, medical facts, epidemiology, and statistics) public health principles (M1, M2)
- Research (preparation for evidence-based clinical practice) (M1 to M4)

- Develop clinical skills and medicalization (physical diagnosis, "introduction to the patient") (M1, M2)
- Exercise clinical skills, develop clinical decision making, experience patient-centered care and shared decision making, technical basic skill development (M3, M4)

The current changing paradigm of medical education—with the compression of basic science and introduction to physical diagnosis and doctor-patient interactions into the first (M1) year; the exercise of clinical skills and introduction to clinical practice in the M2 year; and with fairly open structure for exploring career choices in the M3 and M4 years—will need careful attention to ensure the appropriate development of professional standards and what I call professional socialization, and what others might call "doctoring." Previous attempts to "shorten" the traditional curriculum to three years and truncate the basic science years have met with mixed success. With careful curricular attention to developmentally important aspects and stages of professional medical education, as has been described above, this new paradigm has every chance of success.

We have seen how, for medical education, we need to pay attention to the developmental stages of learners, especially those with the plasticity of "around-twenty-three-year-old" brains. Developmentally and socially, medical students experience rapid but required progression from their first years of basic science, introduction to basic sciences, clinical correlation, and introduction to the patient to, finally, direct patient care as third- and fourth-year medical students. First-year medical students can productively serve and learn as teachers. I have observed many medical students who were very effectively teaching courses on HIV, STDs, and basic health. Middle and high school youngsters are very interested in meeting young medical students from other countries, where both language and introduction to new health policies can be very informative for them. Even college students, while only a little younger, are developmentally much further behind medical students in their maturation. I remember as a college student having two medical students come speak at my fraternity about STDs, contraception, and sexuality. I thought they were so old and mature. They were probably only four years older than I was at the time. I also listened to them more carefully than I would have any "adult."

An exemplary medical student experience was that of Emma Lawrence, a Michigan medical student who, as a University of North Carolina undergraduate, had made several mission trips and had even started a nonprofit to deliver supplies, all to Ghana. When Emma Lawrence came into my office as an aspiring medical student interested in furthering her undergraduate experiences in Ghana, the opportunity to implement and test the professional development pathway and paradigm described above was one that both she and I embraced. As a first-year Michigan medical student, Emma went to Ghana to participate in patient education activities and begin research in electronic fetal monitoring, and she returned to the same hospital as a clinically involved fourth-year medical student demonstrating the developmental paradigm that was outlined above in the discussion of an appropriate professional developmental plan and path. Her story emphasizes once again the importance of bilateral medical student exchanges in our model. They are particularly enhanced when the students from Ghana can meet Michigan students before they go to Ghana, and Michigan students meet students in Ghana before they subsequently come to Michigan, both of which have been experienced by Emma. Her story exemplifies operationally as well as anything the opportunities and strategies I feel are fundamental to an individualized long-view approach to a career in engaged academic global health.

Interview with Doctor Emma Lawrence

Emma Lawrence was a resident in the Obstetrics and Gynecology Department at the University of Michigan from 2015 to 2019. During college at the University of North Carolina as a Morehead-Cain scholar, she founded the NGO MedPLUS Connect to provide equipment, including medical equipment, to rural Northern Ghana. She attended medical school at the University of Michigan and stayed in Ann Arbor for residency, followed by a two-year Global Women's Health fellowship. She received the Velji Leadership Award for Emerging Leaders in Global Health at the 2011 Global Health Conference and Consortium of Universities for Global Health (CUGH) meeting. In 2022 she received funding from the Fogarty International Center for five years to continue her research on hypertension and pregnancy in Ghana. I interviewed her to get her perspective on her global health experiences:

T (Tim Johnson) Emma, you have been doing global health for a long time here at Michigan as a medical student, as a resident. But before you came to Michigan, you were already involved in global health. Can you talk a little bit about your undergraduate experience and how you conceived of what you wanted to do, as I like to say, "What you wanted to be when you grew up," and how you started the NGO that you were involved with?

E (Emma) I went to undergrad at the University of North Carolina. I had the Morehead-Cain scholarship, which had a focus on public service and expanding our global horizons. And so there were different offered experiences during every summer. It encouraged us to experience whatever we were interested in.

And as a high school student, I had spent a couple weeks volunteering in Costa Rica. And that was my first international experience. I was at a school where children were primarily deaf or had other special needs, doing small-scale developmental projects at the school. And that had a huge transformative influence on what I wanted to do going to college. I realized I loved that global engagement, and that made me start thinking about public health.

T So tell me how that high school experience was funded. Did your high school organize it? Who was the organizer of that school?

E [*Laughing*] So my friend and I did a 5K run, when I think we were freshmen in high school, that was helping to support this school in Costa Rica. And so we got interested in that organization. And we asked our parents if we could go during high school if we funded our way. And they said yes. And so we held bake sales for two years, and sold pizza and baked goods at our school. And we made jewelry and bracelets and sold it at our farmer's market and came up with enough money to fund our trip.

T   And how long did you go for?

E   It was like three weeks—in the summer between—I think it was between my junior and senior years of high school.

T   Okay. So you were hooked?

E   Yes. Absolutely.

T   And then, did you apply for this scholarship at UNC? Was it a special opportunity?

E   Yup. It has changed a little bit now, how it's structured, but there were certain high schools that were identified that could each nominate one student who had an interest in global issues and public service. And so I was the nominee from my high school, then there were several rounds of interviews down in North Carolina, and I was selected as one of the students.

T   So you got to North Carolina?

E   Yes. The summer between my first and second year of college is when they funded the global experience, and I wanted to go somewhere new and different. And I had never been to Africa. And Ghana was English-speaking and seemed like a relatively safe and stable place. And so I kind of randomly chose it on a map and then found a program that linked college students with different international health experiences. So I went for two and a half months, so most of my summer was staying with a host family, which was one of my most important criteria when I was looking at these programs. I wanted to live with a local family and have that experience.

And then I was working in an orphanage and doing some outreach, public health work. We were going into local schools. And a lot of the kids would walk to school without shoes and had all these wounds on their feet. So we were working with nurses there and doing basic first aid care.

So that was my first real immersive, "a couple months 'somewhere else'" kind of experience. And then I was totally hooked.

T   That was between your freshman and sophomore years of college?

E   Yup. Absolutely.

T   Okay. So then, after that, what did you do?

E   I felt like this experience was huge for me. I loved Ghana. I formed really close friendships with the people there, including my host family, who I still stay in good touch with. I just had this really incredible summer experience and felt like it had informed what I wanted to do for the rest of my experience in college. And so I wanted other undergrads to have that experience as well.

So for the rest of my summers, I spent at least part of them leading service trips to Ghana. We would take four to six students. I would lead a trip or two a summer for a month each. We would actually go back and stay with that same host family in Kumasi [Ghana] for a couple weeks and then go up north where it's just different, sort of a more rural experience for a couple weeks, and do—

T   And this is the Upper West Region of Ghana?

E   Yup, exactly. And do small projects. And so part of it was the little project we were doing. But the bigger part of it was bringing other students and getting them exposure to a global health experience that I had felt, like, made a big impact in my life and I think makes a big impact. A lot of people decided to go into nursing school or medical school. And that still continues at UNC. And so it's kind of cool. I'm on the LISTSERV [electronic mailing list], and so I see the little projects that they're doing every summer. And they built, you know, pit latrines up in Lawra. They do projects in the orphanage up there.

T   That—Lawra's the village where you've been doing this?

E   Yup. Exactly.

T   From Kumasi to Upper West, that's a pretty big schlep.

E   Yeah.

T   How did you—did you take a bus the first time? Or how did you get up there the first time?

E   Yeah. And again, it was one of those random, serendipitous connections where one of the family friends of the host family in Kumasi was part of a church that had done some service work up north in Lawra and said, "You know, this is a wonderful place with wonderful people. And there's need there. And you guys should check it out." So we got on a *trotro* [a Ghanaian for-hire bus] and took the twelve hours up north and got off the *trotro* there and met Delphina, this lovely woman who we still visit every summer and who cooked us dinner that night, and we have developed relationships with the hospital and the physicians and the orphanage there.

T One of the themes of this book is just this serendipity that you describe.

E Yeah. Oh, yeah.

T The fact that, you know, when you see an opportunity, if it feels safe and it feels right, you should just do it.

E Yeah. Absolutely.

T And kind of unbelievable things happen.

E Yup. Definitely.

T So you got involved in the Upper West.

E Yup.

T And the group that you started at North Carolina was called what?

E It's called Project Heal. So a play on, like, the Tarheels, and then healing: H-E-A-L. Yup, so that continues. And they continue to do projects and lead service trips and fundraisers and all of that. So that's really cool to kind of see undergrads now, like, eight years younger than me, continuing to go back.

T And being involved with that project and kind of leading that project was part of your own leadership development.

E Yeah. Oh, absolutely.

T The Morehead-Cain scholarship program give you a chance to you learn a lot about leadership—

E Absolutely.

T —organization and team building—and team leading.

E Looking back, I was like, I don't know how I did that. What a crazy thing. Like, I was—at that point, a sophomore or junior leading, you know, four or six other undergraduate students, many of whom had never had an international experience, taking them across the globe and traveling this country and being responsible for their mental health and their physical safety and their experience that they had

worked preparing the whole year for. I don't know how their parents
let them come with me.

T   Did you have to convince some of the parents and talk to some of the
parents?

E   Oh, yes, absolutely. I talked to many parents on the phone, many
parents in person. I think we did a really nice job making it as
organized as possible. And it was through—UNC has sort of an
umbrella organization on the campus. And so we had some really
fantastic leadership opportunities. It's the umbrella group for all
their public service organizations. We became part of that. And they
offered really nice mentoring and support. And so we did a nice job,
through collaboration with the leaders who had seen students do stuff
for forever, make sure that our trip seemed structured and reasonable
and safe.

T   Okay. So what else did you do at North Carolina? Did you—was there
another group that you got involved with that was the transporting
equipment group?

E   Yeah. So that was sort of a second offshoot. So at that point,
I had gone back to Ghana probably three summers. And part of the
projects we were doing were bringing basic first aid supplies to some
of the clinics at the school or the clinics up in Lawra. And I was
looking for Band-Aids and gauze and really basic stuff. And so I was
doing some Googling. And I came across MedWish, which is one of
the organizations in Cleveland, which is where I'm from, so again,
serendipitous. And they're one of the supply recovery organizations
that collects huge volumes in their massive warehouse of supplies
from, like, hospitals, clinics, that would otherwise be thrown out.

And so a combination of, you know, a hospital upgrade, and so
their old anesthesia machines that are still functional but no longer,
you know, sync within the hospital, or donated hospital beds when
a hospital upgrades or moves, or lots of new, unopened, unexpired
consumable supplies. When a hospital will no longer order a specific
surgical set. You know, the manufacturer still has hundreds of cartons
on their shelves. And instead of going through the process of trying
to sell that, they just give it to this organization.

So I stumbled across this place in Cleveland looking for Band-Aids. And then at this point, I had built several years of relationships with the physicians at this Lawra district hospital, which is a small, underserved area in northern Ghana, and tried to start making that connection between all these incredible, useful medical supplies we saw sitting in a warehouse in Cleveland, and then the needs of this hospital in Ghana.

And so we got connected with someone who worked for an international shipping company who was from Ghana. He was able to apply, through their philanthropy department, to fund some shipments of supplies to Ghana. We got the supplies donated from this warehouse in Cleveland. We, through him, had the funding covered. We figured out how to navigate with customs, which was quite the ordeal, and got several shipments of supplies to Ghana.

T   And then the containers that went straight to Lawra?

E   Yeah. So the first time, I think it was a couple of pallets full. And then we eventually scaled up to where we were sending containers, like, the back of a semitruck. And then we went to the Ministry of Health and basically said, "We have this track record of over several years, delivering huge volumes of supplies that have a huge value here, make a big impact. Can we partner? And are you interested in helping to fund the cost of shipping supplies to Ghana?" And so that's how the nonprofit was formed, called MedPLUS Connect. So that's something I'm still intimately involved with.

The Project Heal part, the, you know, undergrad students at North Carolina keep doing their thing there. But I'm still involved in MedPLUS. We're still shipping supplies now all throughout northern Ghana, Upper East, Upper West in northern Ghana and to the Northern Region [a populous region south of the Upper East and Upper West regions] to the hospitals that we think have the greatest need, with the Ministry of Health funding the cost of getting supplies there.

T   So MedPLUS has really focused entirely on Ghana?

E   Yeah. Yup. Absolutely.

T   So another thing that I'm writing about is the advice that you should pick one country and focus on it.

E Yeah. Yup. Serendipity and focus. Yeah, absolutely. The number of connections and long-term relationships we have there, we have talked about expanding to other countries. But it's something that would be hard to replicate. The process of—

T Unless you had a whole separate group of people—

E Exactly. Exactly.

T Kind of like what we've done in Ethiopia, right?

E Yup. Yeah. Absolutely.

T We have a whole new group of people who are engaged in a totally different project in Ethiopia. That's country-specific because a lot of it is understanding the country and understanding the culture and understanding what's possible there. And understanding that one country in Africa is different from every other country in Africa.

E Oh, yeah. Absolutely.

T Okay. So that was—so you started a student interest group that travels.

   You started a shipping company. And next, you're applying for medical school?

E Yes.

T And kind of what were you thinking in terms of medical school? Clearly, you're interested in global health.

E Yes.

T Clearly, you're interested in Ghana.

E Yup. Absolutely. Those were two big influences when I was applying to med schools. I applied throughout the country. I interviewed at lots of places that were fantastic, and I felt like I would get a really good education. I had connections in the Ann Arbor area because both of my parents went to undergrad at University of Michigan. My grandparents still lived in Ann Arbor. And I have a really close relationship with them. So when it came down to it, as I was looking at med schools, I felt at any of the schools I was considering I would get a fantastic education and be well prepared for residency, but it was the family connections, the global health connection, the Ghana connection, where I felt like Michigan was just a really good fit.

T Well, as I remember, I think you and I met on your second look. Is that right? Or did we meet on your first look?

E We actually met in my interview. They [the admissions office] recognized that we had a shared interest in Ghana. And they said the two of us have got to meet.

R – my interviewer walked me up to your office because: "You'll never find his office. Let me take you."

T You walked into an office that's like visiting Ghana.

E Yeah. Absolutely. And I was like, this is such a good fit. This is the place for me.

T So tell me a little about what Michigan's global health program, Global REACH, and the fact that there was a global health program meant to you in terms of your decision making.

E The reason I wanted to go to medical school and become a doctor was to have a career where I was engaged in global health. And I, originally throughout undergrad, was planning to go into public health, not medicine. And it was the experiences that I had in Ghana, and then some shadow experiences in a hospital in India, that made me realize I wanted to do medicine and approach global health that way. And so I actually had to do a post-bac [post-baccalaureate] program after undergrad to take my pre-med requirements. That was at Goucher College. They have a specific post-bac program that will let you take all of your classes in one year. It's outside of Baltimore. So I knew when I was doing my search for medical school that that was my number one priority.

Michigan had the specific connection to Ghana, which was such a good fit. But they also had an approach to global health that appealed to me, where it was long-term, sustainable relationships with a small number of countries with students going to those countries, but also local students, residents, faculty coming back to Michigan from the countries. And so I felt that was a really strong fit with the type of global health engagement that I wanted.

T How did you organize your global health experiences? Because medical school is pretty taxing and pretty demanding.

E Yeah.

T   I'll just interject to say that you did exceptionally well in medical school and graduated among the top of your class. But you fit in some global work during school. How, how did you think about how it would fit and where it would fit?

E   When I was starting, I looked ahead to the periods of medical school where there are opportunities to actually leave and go abroad and go back to Ghana. And so the big one was the summer between my first and second year, when we had a couple months off. And I chose to do research in Ghana. And then, a fourth year where there's lots of flexibility, and I was able to spend quite a long time, probably almost three months, in Ghana: a month doing a clinical elective, and then a month and a half doing some research, and then helping two undergraduate students launch their research and get IRB [institutional review board] approval and all of that. I think I had that planned out when I started because I knew I wanted to take all those opportunities to go abroad. And then, when I was here as a medical student, I was a part of the Global Health and Disparities track. And so there were opportunities on a regular basis to stay intellectually involved in global health and discuss articles and be around like-minded students. And then, all the students coming from Ghana, I would always get hooked up with them. And we would cook food and go out. And so I think that engagement was really nice. I got to meet all these people who were my peers and who were medical students in Ghana. And that kind of kept me engaged and excited when I was—

T   And you're still connected with some of them?

E   Oh, absolutely. That's been one of my favorite parts of kind of this journey is that I met—when I was a medical student I met other medical students, both when I was in Ghana and here, and we became—we went through the excitement of becoming doctors together. And then they became house officers, and I became an intern. And we became residents. And we're still friends and now developing into colleagues. And a lot of them have gone into OBGYN. And so now I feel like I have colleagues and friends that I've known for years and years, which is really cool.

T So your medical experience between M1 and M2 year was really research? Had you done research before? Or was that kind of your real first introduction to research?

E That was one of my big, first introductions. As an undergrad, I majored in public policy and psychology. And so I wrote an honors senior thesis through public policy. And it was on the impact of Ghana's new—at that time, new—national health insurance plan. And so I had had some experience doing research in Ghana, but this was the first time it was sort of more of a clinical spin. It was in the hospital. I had a little bit of clinical knowledge, so I could sort of understand what was going on in a hospital setting.

T But it was an opportunity for you to also—to learn about how research was done?

E Oh, absolutely.

T How a hypothesis is developed. And this was at a time when you were also learning about the principles of evidence-based medicine.

E Yes.

T I think that it's appropriate, as you learn how to practice evidence-based medicine to see how the research evidence is collected.

E Mm-hmm.

T And so you had that opportunity to think about how to develop a research study, how to develop a hypothesis, how to collect data, how to analyze data, how to present the data. And the challenges of that, right?

E Yes.

T Research is not always clean and easy.

E Yes. I have a whole new appreciation for doing research in a developing country setting. And it was a great experience. I partnered with a physician in Ghana, so he obviously knew his hospital setting intimately, and then worked with Doctor Frank Anderson here at Michigan, which was great. And I got to be the lead on all steps of the process, of getting IRB [approval] here and there, and the whole data collection, revising our data collection sheet a million times and learning how to analyze the data and all of that. I think that made me realize how interested I was in capacity building and research that evaluated a program and implementation. That was a great experience.

T So how do you think doing that research helped you as you became an M2 and then an M3 year? I mean, you talked about it, doing research in a developing country. Did doing research in a developing country give you insights into research in the United States and, and, the similarities and differences?

E I think that a lot of the steps—whether you're in a developing country or whether you're in the States—a lot of the steps are very similar. The process of going through an IRB is the same. The process of creating a data collection form and being sure to consider issues of picking the right variables in terms of implementation, what that would mean in terms of analyzing the data, it's similar. The sort of analytic skills that you gain in terms of understanding the research that you're doing and doing the statistics and being able to read other people's papers is the same, and the process of writing up something that's academic and publishable is the same. So I think almost all the skills are very transferable.

T Okay. So, research between your M1 and your M2 year. And then in M4, you went over again. And at this point, you had taken "Introduction to the Patients." You'd already taken clinical skills classes. And you had done all your clinical clerkships, including OBGYN.

E Yup.

T So you were ready to be kind of an active subintern, as we often describe the M4 years. And you were able to help the residents and other doctors take care of patients and actually do clinical care and do operations, when you were—over there as an M4. Is that right?

E Yup. Yeah.

T So how—tell me about that. This is a foreign country, where you started as a sophomore in college. And dreamed about what you could do, thinking it would be public health. Suddenly, now, you're actually almost a doctor, helping to operate on patients and putting your hands into people's abdomens and delivering babies.

E Yeah. Yeah. Yup.

T Tell me about that.

E That was really incredible. I think that was one of my favorite experiences in Ghana. It was towards the end of my M4 year. And so I was—I knew I was doing OBGYN. I had already applied. I was waiting for match day. And I was almost at the point of being a physician. And so I spent a little over a month doing a clinical elective. And I was just fully integrated with other medical students at my level there.

T And this is in Kumasi, where you'd already worked before?

E This was in Kumasi. So I'd spent a long time there previously. I knew the hospital well. I knew a lot of the attendings previously. I actually knew a lot of the medical students because either they had come to Michigan or I had met them on previous trips. And I, you know, lived in the dorms with the medical students. And we, you know, we ate our lunches together and walked to the hospital together. And I lived my life for those four or five weeks as a medical student there with them, which was fantastic. I felt like the experience was challenging from a clinical perspective, but also very much, as you said, at my level. And so I got to first assist on C-sections. I got to deliver babies. I got to go through the process of thinking about patients and plans and assessments. And so really got involved in a clinical sense there, which was fantastic and was a really good preparation for being an intern, which I was a couple months after that.

T We know in Ghana, they don't have the technical equipment that we have here. How did being in Ghana emphasize the importance of physical exam and history taking and having to be very selective in getting labs and having to wait a long time for certain things? How did that—how did that affect your becoming a doctor?

E It makes you think much more critically about what you're ordering and why. And I think that was particularly helpful starting as an intern, when there are three million tests available that you can order on any patient. And then revisiting that recently when I went back, now with a year and a half of being a resident under my belt. Their clinical exam skills are fantastic, and it makes me realize how much we rely on ultrasound for fetal position, on how much we rely on all of our tests to see if a patient is sick or not. And they have a really, sort of fine-tuned assessment of whether a patient is sick or not by just looking at them, by feeling their belly.

And when they order a test, the patient literally has to pay out of pocket then, which often means the patient getting on their cell phone, calling the family member. The family member coming in with the fifteen cedis [at the time, about fifteen cents], just enough that they can gather up for that one test, going to the lab, getting it done, getting it back, and then maybe ordering another one.

When I was in Ghana recently, there was a patient who was really sick from a septic abortion. And she had no family with her. On rounds, we literally went around in a circle, and all the medical students and residents each gave ten cedis [about two dollars] or so, so she could go get an ultrasound and a CBC. And so—

T   So that's a lot of money there.

E   Yeah, exactly. Right. Here—and here, you don't think about it. You just click on all the labs, and everyone gets them every morning. And you get them done, and they come back. And often, they aren't fundamental key making of medical decisions. So I think we're fortunate, and our patients are fortunate to get care and to practice here, where we have so many resources. But it does really make you think about what you need to have to provide good care to a patient.

T   Yeah. I remember one time when I saw that the residents actually carried suture. And if patients couldn't afford suture, they would do the operations with "their suture," and then afterwards, before the patients could be discharged, they or their family would have to replace the suture.

E   Yup. Yup. It's incredible. It's incredible what the hospital is able to do and the physicians are able to do with so little.

T   Okay. So, graduated from medical school. You walked across the stage. You're now Doctor Lawrence.

E   Yup. Yay.

T   And you started residency, which is even more busy and, and even more crazy than medical school, especially internship. [The first year of training after medical school, "first year of residency" is the preferred language. "Intern" is a term that was used at the time when graduates just of out of medical school had to actually live full time in the hospital for the first year.]

Tell me about kind of how you planned and how you executed your Ghana experience as a resident. What kind of experiences you wanted to get out that were resident experiences, not medical student experiences.

E   So part of it was definitely knowing I wanted to do more research and more clinical research and trying to get involved in that, because that's something that I could do while I was here. And connection with folks in Ghana, understanding that, you know, throughout my whole intern year, there were no opportunities to go abroad. And then in the second year, [it] was taking the opportunities I did have to get back to Ghana, now as a doctor, with many more sort of practical, clinical skills. And so for my elective time in my second year, I was able to go back to Ghana for close to a month. I actually went to Accra this time. Yes. So I had spent a lot of clinical time in Kumasi, and so this time, figured I would go to the other big hospital and spend some clinical time there. And the other reason I went to Accra is I'm working on developing a research project on duration of magnesium sulfate for women who have severe preeclampsia or eclampsia. And the physician there who I am collaborating with is the current chief resident in Accra. He is also a trained clinical pharmacologist.

T   Okay.

E   He's a very smart guy. And he had spent time here at Michigan. And so we met in Ann Arbor there and sat in his room in the ICC [Inter-Cooperative Council, where many of the visiting Ghana students and residents stay] and talked about the research while he was here. And then, we and other colleagues sort of worked on it independently when he was in his second-to-last year of residency and I was an intern. And then I went as an HO2 [second-year house officer or resident] when he was a chief resident a year later to start working on actually implementing things.

T   So how was Accra different than Kumasi?

E   Kumasi will always have a special place in my heart. I love Kumasi. Accra is bigger. Accra is a little more like the academic hospitals in the Global North. The hospital itself is similar to KATH. It's a little bit better resourced. Everything is slightly newer. I think there's a little bit more of a focus on research, and the residents have a little more supportive resources when it comes to research. But, I mean, OBGYN is the same, the same issues in Kumasi as it is in Accra. They have the same sort of limitations when it comes to resources. And the pathology [severity of the cases seen] is more advanced, but it's the same things we see here in Michigan, which is one of the things I love so much about OBGYN. Yes, they have their sickle cell, and we have our patients with lupus. But, but, like, 99 percent of it, it's the same problems. And we do the same things. And it was really fun to be back there as a resident and to now have residents who are my peers and colleagues and having the same conversations that I would have with residents here, trying to work through patient cases. So you would be in the labor room. And it would be 2 a.m. and a Korle Bu resident would be there, and I would be there. And the attendings are sleeping. And something happens and we're talking through and trying to figure out what to do. So that was really cool.

T   So now, you're finishing your second year of residency. What's the plan for, for the rest of the time?

E   Next year, hopefully back to Ghana to follow up on the research that we're doing. I've realized now, from past research experiences, that nothing happens quickly. So we're in the final processes of getting IRB approval. We have our data collection forms going and sort of piloted there. But it's going to take at least a year to collect enough data. That will be something that I hope I'll get to spend a lot of time on the next two years. And then, ultimately, I'm thinking very strongly about doing one of the fellowships in global health. I think clinically, I want to be a generalist. I love obstetrics. I love gynecology, at least in this point unless something drastic happens. I can't imagine giving up any of it. And so I think my sort of focus or specialization will be global health. And Ghana is my country. As it is yours. I want to continue to go back and have that engagement and work on projects in capacity building, and then, research that evaluates the impact of those projects.

T Still interested in the public health—

E Yeah.

T —and public policy questions that you were interested in as an undergraduate. So, so there's a theme, and there's also an arc.

E Definitely.

T So—anything you would do differently?

E Oh, that's a good question. I think so much of what I've done since an undergrad was just kind of stumbling into things that interested me and relationships that I developed. And I just sort of went with it. It's not like I knew when I was twelve years old that this was my plan or trajectory. And I think it changes along the way. So I think I've just kind of gone with it.

T But there's been intentionality as well.

E Yeah.

T A combination of opportunity and intentionality.

E Yup. That's true. That's very true.

T We talked earlier about public policy and public health.

E Yeah.

T Any regrets about doing medicine?

E No. Absolutely not.

T Why do you think medicine was the right career choice for you?

E I think part of it is, I get—I just enjoy it. I love interacting with patients. I get a lot of personal fulfillment about that person-to-person, hands-on—doing a C-section and handing someone their baby is the most incredible feeling ever. I also think that if you want to do public health, understanding medicine, understanding the clinical sides of things, understanding what needs to happen on the ground for a hospital to run is incredibly important. I think it's hard, if you're doing public health and you don't grasp that sort of clinical aspect, to really do a good job that does meaningful change.

Lessons Learned

Introduce global health early to receptive health care learners.

Opportunity and intentionality are both important.

Think about the developmental stages of learners.

Attention must be paid to the ethical parameters of global medical and health programs.

Chapter 7

Faculty Career Development: Academics, Research, and Leadership

Faculty development has been integral in the program from its inception. Early on, many of the Ghanaians I met (e.g., Doctor Amoa) had traveled to Hopkins for faculty development courses that focused on teaching and research skills as well as leadership training. From the very beginning stages of the GPTP, developing faculty was an intentional and important part of the training. The Ghana Management Committee's continued predominance was paired with a desire for Ghanaian faculty to continuously increase their academic advancement. They participated in all aspects of program development and implementation. From the educational perspective, many of the curricular material, slide sets, teaching packs, and eventually, PowerPoint slides were handed off to the Ghanaians by the professors from the United Kingdom and United States so that they could then take up and take over the teaching load. Luckily, there were several senior, long-serving faculty members who could serve as faculty development mentors and advisors. This included Doctor Joseph Martey and his few senior colleagues in Kumasi, including Doctor Sidney Adadevoh, who had previously done a faculty sabbatical funded by the Fogarty International Center at Michigan, and senior faculty in Accra, led by Doctors J. B. Wilson, K. K. Korsah, Ghosh and others. But not only could they provide faculty guidance and advice to junior faculty, they were also interested in faculty development for their own careers. When Professor Cecil Klufio returned from Papua New Guinea, he was able to become very actively involved in these efforts and serve not only as mentor but also role model with his international presentations and regular publications, including a book on research statistics (Klufio, 2003).

Faculty development included not only engagement in terms of curriculum, teaching, and teaching skills but also in scholarship and academics. How to do research, research design, and publication were all part of the training. Early on, research of the senior residents often included faculty, and these papers were published in the *Ghana Medical Journal*, regional African journals, the *International Journal of Gynecology and Obstetrics*, and occasionally even major "high-impact" international journals. As has been highlighted several times, peer-review publication was always an intentional priority of the leaders of the GPTP for publication and dissemination of program descriptions and evaluations and of the research being conducted by faculty, fellows, residents, and students under the umbrella of GPTP and beyond. The first report on the GPTP was presented and published by Professor Cecil Klufio, with a Ghanaian first author, two more Ghanaian coauthors, and three out of the five authors were Ghanaian. That action was well received and was recognized by many within the GPTP. This intention for shared authorship on publications became a policy to have local coauthors on all publications (and presentations, posters, etc.). This probably led, in no small part, to the textbooks that were published (Kwawukume & Emuveyan, 2002, 2005), being entirely African authored, African edited, and African published. These publications and presentations were important to advance the academic careers of local faculty, but the policy also insured that research data and intellectual property were not "stolen" from Ghanaian authors or institutions. It also ensured that foreign researchers identified and included local colleagues at the very conception phase of the research project. These principles of "community-based participatory research" were ingrained from the inception in the GPTP and were emphasized in the Charter documents (Chapter 8; Kekulawala & Johnson, 2018; Spector-Bagdady & Johnson, 2021). Doctor Adanu and I were on the editorial board of the *International Journal of Gynecology and Obstetrics*, the official journal of FIGO, when it adopted a similar policy for its publications: "local co-authors will be included as a policy on all papers from LMIC to support (FIGO) priorities for capacity building as well as to prevent co-opting of research by high income countries" (Adanu et al., 2017). This policy of required local coauthorship in publications from LMIC is becoming a more common and widely adopted editorial policy among many journals (Adanu et al., 2017; Spector-Bagdady & Johnson, 2021).

In addition to scholarly publications, as we have already seen, publication of books was important, and the first was *Comprehensive Obstetrics in the Tropics*, which was edited by Yao Kwawukume and E. Ejiro Emuveyan with all West African authors. This book was reviewed in the *Lancet* (Olatunbosun, 2002) and provided not only evidence of scholarship and academics but also gave a textbook to residents and medical students so that they could study and understand and learn what was expected for their examinations. It was a major innovation that there were textbooks that matched the curriculum, and teachers told learners what they were expected to learn and know, a very American approach. These textbooks were published locally, entirely by faculty members, and were readily available for between the equivalent of twenty and thirty dollars, which was much less than the several hundred dollars for hardcover European or American textbooks, and therefore they became standard use for Ghanaian learners at all levels.

In addition, small, inexpensive students' handbooks were written and published locally by Doctor Joseph Seffah and others. The initial textbook in obstetrics was followed by a textbook in gynecology, and subsequently a textbook in family planning, which was written entirely by the family planning fellows with faculty support, and so an early entrée to scholarly writing and publication for them. The family planning text was modeled on the *Johns Hopkins Manual of Gynecology and Obstetrics*, which has always been authored as an educational and career development exercise by the OBGYN residents overseen by the faculty at Johns Hopkins (Johnson, Hallock et al., 2015). Evidence of scholarship and textbook publication were an important part of faculty development. Obviously, their research skills led to the success of many. Doctor Richard Adanu, whom we shall shortly hear from, went on to get an MPH at Johns Hopkins and was a successful faculty member and then dean of the University of Ghana School of Public Health. He followed me as the editor-in-chief of the *International Journal of Gynecology and Obstetrics* (IJGO), having been brought on by me to the editorial board when I was editor as an associate editor responsible for editing some of the subsections. Richard also was very involved in the early days of the Ethiopian project described below, where the desire for research methodology by the Ethiopian faculty members as the residency developed was satisfied by African South-to-South engagement—one of the key aspirations for developing LMIC academic programs. Richard provided the early research education and teaching to the Ethiopians and continues to travel to Ethiopia on a regular basis for research teaching.

So faculty development was really something that happened from academic institution to academic institution. While JHIEPGO and other NGOs had done faculty training and used academic faculty to do it, I do think the true university-to-university partnership of the Ghana Postgraduate Training Programme assisted interested national professional societies and institutions in providing a high-quality level of faculty development to the long-term success and development of the faculty members in Ghana and subsequently, as we shall see, to the long term faculty development of faculty members at St. Paul's Hospital Millennium Medical College in Ethiopia (Chapter 10).

Faculty development includes teaching development, pedagogy development, and curriculum development along with high-quality multiuse teaching materials such as PowerPoint slides, which quickly replaced the glass slides of the early days of the program after the introduction of personal computers and soon, access to the internet. Academic research, scholarship, publication of clinical articles and development from case reports to clinical trials to translational research and, ultimately, health services research, outcomes research, and hopefully, implementation science in the future are aspirational goals across the academy (Peterson et al., 2011, 2018). This shows a natural progression of the types of academic research and scholarship we can expect in low-income countries as they develop academic capacity. Current students, such as those interested in clinical pharmacology, are going to be doing basic science and translational research as well. Faculty development in Ghana was very important, and successful productivity has led to promotion and recognition, with faculty moving up the academic ranks to deanships and ultimately starting their own medical schools, as Doctor Kwawukume, who was a resident at the initiation of the GPTP, has successfully demonstrated with Family Health University College Medical School.

To give a view of the approach taken in the GPTP to faculty development, I interviewed Doctor Richard Adanu.

Interview with Professor (Rector) Richard Adanu

Richard Adanu is the former dean of the School of Public Health at the University of Ghana and current rector of the Ghana College of Physicians and Surgeons. A graduate of the University of Ghana Medical School (UGMS), he completed his residency in obstetrics and gynecology at KBTH in Accra as part of the Carnegie Postgraduate Training Program. He did a senior resident rotation at the University of Michigan and identified as a goal a career in public health. After returning to the faculty of obstetrics and gynecology at UGMS and after qualifying for the West African College of Surgeons, he obtained a Gates Fellowship, which supported him to complete an MPH at Johns Hopkins as a member of Delta Omega, the public health honor society. Initially returning to the obstetrics and gynecology faculty at UGMS, he turned a part-time appointment in the Department of Population, Family, and Reproductive Health in the School of Public Health into a full-time appointment, and ultimately, appointment as dean at the age of forty-four. He is a FWACS, FGCS, honorary FACOG, and immediate past editor of the *International Journal of Gynecology and Obstetrics* (IJGO), the official journal of FIGO. In 2022 he was elected to the US National Academy of Medicine of the National Academies of Science.

T (Tim Johnson) Richard, when did you finish your training in OBSTGYNAE as part of the Ghana Postgraduate Training Programme?

R (Richard Adanu) I finished in 2001 [giving a start date of 1996].

T When did you first hear about the Ghana Postgraduate Training Programme?

R I think the first time I heard it must have been in 1995, when I was doing my house officer job. [The required one to two years of hospital experience for all Ghana medical school graduates before entering practice, six months each in OBGYN, internal medicine, pediatrics and surgery. Also called "houseman job."] I was doing my six-month house job in OBGYN after medical school. We house officers knew that there was a postgraduate training program going on in the department. The one thing we talked a lot about was how the department was turning out consultants faster than the other three major departments, Internal Medicine, Surgery, and Pediatrics. So that was when everybody was telling us about this special program, together with telling us about the possibility of doing it.

T Did you always think you wanted to do OBST and GYNAE?

R Well, I actually didn't want to do OBST and GYNAE. As much as I enjoyed the rotation, I mean, I was working with Doctor Ghosh [Doctor T. S. Ghosh was an Indian who trained in India and served as a sponsored Commonwealth consultant in Ghana for almost his entire career. He was a beloved surgical teacher and academic mentor.] I really didn't want to do OBSTGYNAE. I wanted to do community health and epidemiology, my mates thought that was kind of like, crazy. So after I finished my houseman job I couldn't get placement for community health, so then I came back and say, "Hey, I mean, I'll do OBSTGYNAE." So that's how I got into the program.

T But you were always interested in epidemiology and primary care?

R Yeah, always.

T So you started the OBGYN training program, and then at some point, I think you came to Ann Arbor for a rotation during the last year.

R Yeah, that was in 2000.

T So as you were doing the residency, did you see kind of a new direction forming for your career in obstetrics and gynecology?

R I think at the time of the residency, I really didn't see that way. Because during a busy residency with all the training, my mind was that I was going to go on this clinical path. But I think coming to Ann Arbor and meeting people like—I think Vanessa Dalton [now professor of obstetrics and gynecology and associate chair for research in the UM OBGYN Department] was in her final year of residency then, and she had an MPH already. And then seeing people on the faculty who had, who held combined MDs and MPHs, that got me thinking, realizing that it wasn't impossible. As much as I saw the public health aspects in what we're doing. But I think the time that—it was three months in Ann Arbor—kind of like shaped it for me, that I would definitely like to do public health in combination with OBGYN, and I think we talked about it.

T Yeah, I think—I asked the usual question I ask, which was: "What do you want to be when you grow up?" and you said you were interested in doing epidemiology. When you came to Ann Arbor, you really came with your long commentary and your short commentaries [written research summaries and case summaries required for the Part 2 final examination of the West African College of Surgeons] so you could complete them and to see what medicine was like in our high-income environment and to prepare for the Part 2 written and oral examinations. What was your long commentary on?

R My long commentary, OB one, was on ruptured uterus. It was a five-year retrospective review of ruptured uterus cases. And then the GYNAE one was on knowledge and practice of cervical cancer screening amongst Ghanaian women.

T So they were both kind of epidemiology related?

R Yeah, they were, yeah. And I hoped to get both of them published [see Adanu & Obed, 2001; Adanu, 2004].

T   So then, you went back to Ghana and took the exams and passed. Congratulations. And then I think that what you were told, that if you were a good junior faculty member and if you were to teach and continue to be successful academically, that there might be other opportunities. What did you go back thinking you were going to do long term?

R   Well, when I went back—I mean, I think you and I have talked about the whole public health thing. And I think at that time I said, "Well, do we have the opportunity at the Ghana School of Public Health?" I think you advised me that it might be advisable to get further education outside Ghana so that if we could get into Johns Hopkins or to Michigan, that would preferable.

T   I think we targeted Hopkins.

R   Yeah. We targeted Hopkins first, yeah. That would be helpful. So when I went back at that time, when I left Michigan with the mindset that the first option was doing public health in addition to OBGYN. And my second option was to go into urogynecology and not the public health side of things, because I spent quite some time with John Delancey [a prominent urogynecologist and gynecologic surgeon] when I was out in Michigan. So then, I got back and there was talk about subspecialty training, which was going on then, but these were the two options in my mind. So I went back, did the GREs [Graduate Record Examination, generally required for admission to schools of public health] and got admission to Hopkins. It was probably at the same time, in 2003, Hopkins gave me admission, then I got onto the UGMS faculty, but I didn't go in 2003 because of a delay in getting the scholarship.

T   I think we hooked you up with Bernie Guyer [Professor Bernie Guyer, chair of the Department of Maternal and Child Health at Johns Hopkins Bloomberg School of Public Health] who I knew well and—did you get to meet him in Ghana?

R   Yeah. I met Bernie Guyer in Ghana before I came to Hopkins in 2004.

T   He was doing some kind of a research site visit?

R   Yeah. He had a partnership with the University of Ghana School of Public Health. So after I got the admission, then Bernie came down for a meeting in Accra.

T And he saw how capable you were. The rest was kind of history with you. I mean, you went to Hopkins. You thrived, despite the fact that your family, a wife and three children, stayed in Ghana. You came back to Ghana and joined the medical school faculty.

R Yeah. I took a leave to go to Hopkins, but I came back and rejoined faculty.

T But then shortly thereafter, had an appointment in the School of Public Health.

R Yeah. So when I came back to Accra—

T With an MPH.

R Yeah, with an MPH. I was up teaching in the OBGYN Department and the Community Health Department. So I was doing those two with the medical school.

T So they—community health was in the medical school? [In sub-Saharan Africa, it is often the schools of public health.]

R It was part of the medical school then. And then I think about a few months after that, I started doing part-time teaching, also at the School of Public Health.

T And that's in MCH?

R Yeah, in MCH. That was like 2006. So then, I was doing all this at the same time, until 2010 December, when I did a transfer from the OBGYN Department to the School of Public Health.

T And then that became kind of more of a permanent thing.

R Yeah. It became more of a permanent thing. So since 2010, I no more teach the residents and the medical students in OBGYN. I mean, it's more of like teaching the graduate students and the family planning fellows, I mean, the ones [subspecialist trainees] from Accra all come and do the Public Health school. And I get to advise some of them.

T And the ones in Kumasi...?

R The ones in Kumasi enter the KNUST Department of Community Medicine for their advanced degree. Now they do the MPH also, yeah. But I still kind of like to do some clinical practice at Legon hospital, not the teaching hospital, the service side of the future teaching hospital.

T So tell me about what you have done since going full time in the School of Public Health at the University of Ghana. Since then, your career has really blossomed, so what kinds of things in the last seven years have you taken on, in addition now to being dean of the School of Public Health?

R   Well, the first thing that was the *International Journal of Gynecology and Obstetrics*, that started in—back in 2006, right as I finished the MPH.

T   And I think you were working on Contemporary—

R   "Contemporary Issues" ["Contemporary Issues" is one of the monthly features in IJGO], yeah. I did that first with you, then later with three others, including Doctor Vincent Boama, who I met when we were sponsored fellows at the FIGO Congress in Kuala Lumpur. Then, in 2014, got appointed editor-in-chief of the journal. Another line that has developed is collaboration with WHO's Reproductive Health and Research unit. I started out with just being a temporary advisor in one of their meetings.

T   How did that happen?

R   What happened was that there was one student of mine, one student from Hopkins who I co-supervised because she came down to do her PhD data collection in Ghana. Then, after she finished her PhD, she introduced me to the WHO Reproductive Health and Research staff that were interested in research similar to some of our things. So then, I had a temporary—an advisory role. Then we collaborated on projects, and currently I regularly participate in all their meetings to determine policy among their scientific technical advisory group and also on their guidelines developing a group for maternal health. There is another line I've been collaborating with other universities. So the University of Southampton, NYU, these are the main ones, and then there are a few others—the School of Public Health is collaborating with them.

T   And what are your South-South partners?

R   South-South partners. We have Ethiopia.

T   And—actually, you went to Ethiopia as the kind of—to kick off the research program there.

R   Yeah. So that's—there's that one thing that's going on. There's an ongoing partnership with St. Paul [see Chapter 9]. I mean, it started off with a research capacity-building workshop, then I began doing some research for their faculty, and that has been going on every year. I go there whenever the academic programs want to do some research training. They actually invited me the last year to examine OBGYN residents, and I think I'm going to be doing that for three years before then they have to get a new person. And then there's also—in Nigeria there's University of Ibadan with whom I am linked with NYU. There's a training that we do for residents and clinical faculty, research training. And Nigeria also has a WHO—a participating center. That is true, a collaborating center: one project we are doing now, looking at abortion complications, where we are one center for the study and Ibadan is also a center for that study. So there are many things I've entered into as a result of this collaboration.

T I want to go back to the Ghana Postgraduate Training Programme. Clearly, you're one of the great successes of the program. But I guess I wonder, how do you think the program helped you specifically?

R I think the program helped me in the sense that I managed to see more than just what the Ghanaian context could offer, because we had faculty members from the US, faculty members from the UK come in to do guest lectures, revision programs, and clinical teaching. Internationally-known specialists came for the revisions.

T You were there in the early years of the program?

R Yeah. So I saw the perspective of other people. So core faculty and management team was based in Ghana, the training was kind of like, international, because you saw the different approach coming from the US and different approach of who's coming from the UK, then the Ghanaian faculty also. The program also helped us through the funding, like, we had learning resources in the department library. We had the *British Journal of Obstetrics and Gynaecology* from UK, and we had the *International Journal [of Gynecology and Obstetrics]*, and we had the Green Journal [*Obstetrics and Gynecology*] from the US. And we had current issues of those journals. So that kind of like, made that feel very much in touch with them.

T Back before the days of internet and World Wide Web.

R   Exactly. Long before the days of the internet. Everybody has access
    now, yes, with smartphones, yeah. So that really helped then. Then
    there was—

T   That was 2000 and—

R   So this was like—I entered the training—I did my primaries in 1996,
    so I entered the program kind of like in 1997.

T   So back in those days, you had to do a primary examination that was
    the basic science qualifying entrance examination.

R   Yeah. And two years after that, the Part 1.

T   The entry exam and that was very much based on the British system.
    The British emphasized basic science knowledge more than the
    American system.

R   Yeah, yeah.

T   So compare and contrast what you think the British added and the
    Americans added to the program.

R   I think the British basically came in more with the UK perspective
    and training—many of our consultants had trained in the UK—and
    then they also came in bringing in a bit of emphasis on independence.
    You had to read extensively. The Americans came and brought in
    structure. It's like, with the UK system, while you're preparing for
    your exams and you are on your own, but with the US system, you're
    not on your own. You've got to get this done in five years. So I'll tell
    you that's kind of like the main difference that we saw. And probably
    from the American side also; I think at that time the British are not
    so much into medical-legal issues and patient-centered care, want the
    patient's opinion, dialoging with the patient. We got that more from
    the US faculty.

T   So when you were a resident, it was pretty much Ghanaian faculty.

R   It was.

R   Many people had come out, I mean Kwawukume [Yao Kwawukume,
    early Accra grad, eventual department head at KBTH, and founding
    president of the Family Health Medical School], Seffah [Joseph
    Seffah, UGMS faculty who was important in the uptake of ultrasound
    and management of intrauterine growth restriction], Obed [Samuel
    Obed, who went on to become department head and CEO of

KBTH], Kwabena Danso [early KATH graduate, eventual chair and medical school dean of KNUST], they all got out early. So they were the early, early graduates and successes.

T So they were really Ghanaian early graduates and leaders.

R They were Ghanaians.

I They had taken advantage of the American and the British and the Ghanaian mixture, but—

R But by the time we were finishing, I mean, these were people who had gone through the same program that we are going through, who were now on faculty and were examiners with the college. And actually, Kwawukume was, he was head of department at the time at Korle Bu. He was a program graduate and already was head of the department at the time that I graduated here.

T And so would it be fair to say that by the time you graduated, pretty much the program was a Ghanaian-taught and -directed program?

R It was. It was. By the time I graduated it had its own identity and its own structure. But then we still had viable linkages, probably more with the US than the UK.

T And those are ongoing relationships, right? I think Michigan and a couple places in the UK were pretty much the only places—

R Yeah. It was Michigan then, pretty much. Earlier on, people have gone to LSU with Doctor Tom Elkins and then Hopkins, when he moved there, then with Doctor Jim Blythe, some people had gone to St. Louis.

T And then with Doctor Jack Sciarra at Northwestern. But I think the comment you made about by 2001, 2002, it really had a Ghanaian identity, which it continues to have now.

My next question is: Why do you think it worked in Ghana? It worked for you so—well, why did it work for you?

R Well, it worked for me because I would say there were examples I had—I mean, it's probably different for everyone, but I saw people who had gone through the program, who had finished, and who were getting onto faculty within the medical school. So that, to me, kind of like showed that there was a future. Unlike other departments, where there were people who were residents when we were medical students, and we were finished with our residency before some of them. And so you could see that there was a future, you could pass exams and get on faculty and have a career.

T   I think that idea of progressing regularly through a program is an American one; move on, progression, get through the program.

R   Exactly. And it wasn't only—they weren't only on faculty in the medical school. There were people who moved out of Accra, who moved to the Central Region of the country and Northern Region. Dr Addo-Tagoe became, like, a country director for, I think it was Engender Health [an NGO]. It was somebody like one of the graduates, Doctor Amo-Mensah, who moved into the medical services of the Police Service—it's more like they [Ghana Health Service, MOH, university administration] send you to the most prominent institution and a hospital with just one specialist, and you became the consultant in charge. So you saw people getting into academic medicine, into practice, and into things like public health, agency work, public planning, that kind of thing, so there were career prospects. So that was definitely very encouraging. So that was one thing that made it work. The other thing that made it work was probably linked to the confidence that what you were doing in your medical practice was right. You didn't need to necessarily have some extra foreign or international training. And I think what did that was the three months of placement abroad, where you see everything that's being done and you're able to kind of like compare work being done and how you can place that in the context with what you're doing and kind of like know that what you're doing is not wrong, it is contextualized. And being able to sit in meetings with residents and attendings, say, in or from the US, having discussions with them and knowing that what you say is correct [in terms of clinical management]. I mean, kind of like, let's grow some confidence in what we are teaching medical students and all that. The fact that there was probably a progression, and there was also the fact that when you were teaching, you knew that you could achieve success. That helped and—the international collaboration.

T   So why do you think this program was so successful in Ghana?

R Well, I think the program was successful, one, because the Ghanaian residents, the Ghanaian faculty then didn't have another place to go to, which might not seem like the best reason to create a big program, but things got to the state where the [Ghana] government was not going to send anybody to the UK.

T And the UK wasn't going to accept anybody.

R And the US would not accept anybody. It was literally impossible to get into an OBGYN residence in the US. So people had to get something to work in Ghana. Now, if at that time it was only the Ghanaian faculty, maybe the determination would have been there to set it up, because there are departments, such as the surgery department, which were in the same situation. But then having the support of the Royal College [RCOG] and then the American College and saying, "Let's build this with the Carnegie funding," that, I think, then got people to develop it. And we also went in with trust.

There were candidates who were still trying to see how they could get to the UK or whatever. By the time we came in, we knew that this was not going to be possible.

So I think that's partly that the circumstances were just right. Because if there had still been the opportunity going to the UK they would have moved out to the UK.

T But basically now, I mean, since 1990s there have been no opportunities for anybody in any country in Africa to get outside of the continent, not from Ethiopia, not from Kenya, not from Uganda, right?

R I mean, people still go, but they go as individuals and—it's not a program that is sending them. It was like this college program sends you, found a place for you, and you have your training. But now, these things are uncommon.

T Now it's a "golden lottery" ticket.

R Yeah. It is.

T But you've been pretty successful.

R Yes, I have.

T Any regrets?

R No regrets at all. I mean, this I had to do to get the training I wanted, I would still do it the same way. The reason I'm saying this is that some of my mates who came to the UK when almost nobody went—did OBGYN in the US, they came to the UK and did OBGYN, and the truth is that the opportunities that I have, the committees that I sit on, the importance of things that I speak to, many of them, although we kind of finished at the same time, they don't get those opportunities. I guess it's because they are in the UK. There are quite many people there who can be seen as experts. But had they been in Ghana. That gives, kind of like—that opens the door for an international invitation, which a Ghanaian in the UK wouldn't be invited to. There are a number of them that I have talked with who say that, but the truth is I have no regrets about it all.

T Well, I mean, a lot of people have had a successful pathway. I mean, you have had a successful pathway in public health. Obed has had a successful pathway in administration. Seffah, a successful pathway in clinical teaching. People have found success in the Ghana College and the West African College. Because the other interesting thing is, the program was started to train people from the West African College, and the Ghanaian College was kind of an unexpected development. I don't know if you know it yet, but in 2016, forty people all took the membership exams for the Ghana College in OBSTGYNAE, and I understand all forty of them passed; now you're really starting to see a waterfall effect.

R Definitely. And probably close to 90 percent of the teachers and the examiners are products of the Ghana Postgraduate Training Programme.

T I don't know if you heard, but Emma [Emmanuel] Morhe is going as inaugural head of department to the new school, UHAS, in Ho.

R I am not surprised. He's got credible publications and an MPH. And there's Kolbilla [Doctor David Kolbilla, a KNUST grad and family planning and reproductive health fellowship, which included an MSc, MPH equivalent, who was head of department and is now Tamale Teaching Hospital CEO] at UDS in Tamale. And Doctor Joseph Adu, who is a well-respected OBGYN educator at the University of Cape Coast. So we have people everywhere across the country.

T Well, what other things do you have to say about the Ghana Postgraduate Training Programme?

R The training that we had also has allowed many to contribute the knowledge in terms of publications, because the wave of promotion within the university was by research productivity and academic output. So there's more of a desire to contribute to knowledge with the OBGYN faculty than I see in many of the others [departments]. It's been that way for a long time. The Ghana program started in 1989, that's when I was getting into medical school. It has been such a strong program. It has been. But I think many of the other programs have developed from the GPTP model, like emergency medicine, family medicine, ENT, which has got a good program now.

There are many things that are important to remark on: the benefit has not only been OBGYN. There's been OBGYN successes, and it is expanding to the new medical schools in Ghana, after OBGYN have come these other programs. OBGYN really was a role model locally, and then it's grown even outside the country now to Ethiopia and expanded.

Yeah. So the effect has gone beyond the OBGYN practice in the country, and I think that's the thing that we should always mention. Because it started at that single specialty, but then it kind of like gave rise to other specialty training.

T So being in public health, can you talk a little bit about, kind of the public health benefits of the OBGYN program? One of the critiques of the program really is why should you train specialists when the country needs kind of to have more general doctors and health care workers. Have you seen downstream public health benefits from training OBGYN specialists in Ghana?

R I think—I mean, when we look at things like mortality figures, child mortality figures have improved over the years in the country. From OBGYN, like, there's Doctor Ernest Maya, who is also on faculty at our school, he has grown so much into public health training. That's one of the things he does. He's like a trainer and an examiner for the medical training school.

So Maya goes around training midwives. Those are public health benefits. Midwives are the ones who kind of like take the majority of births in Ghana. Now these midwives are having graduates of our GPTP impacting their training so that we come out kind of like—they have multiplied what they are doing. You think of family planning: Ghana's family planning contraceptive prevalence is probably not as high as we would like it to be, but then the family planning fellows are running the different LARC [long-acting reversible contraceptive] training centers. We are working with the Ghana health centers. We are contributing to health policy. We are training midwives in family planning and practices. So there have been this kind of things that have come out just from this training. Because you can't get maternal and child health going without obstetricians at the forefront. If you don't train obstetricians to lead and develop policies, you wouldn't have the impact; there wouldn't be generational change because the midwives would just do their practice, most of them, and then get on, but these new obstetricians are raising up the next generations of midwives, generations of obstetricians. So the long-term effect, the population effect, is big.

Lessons Learned

Develop and support academic leaders.

The basics of faculty development are universal and replicable.

It is good to have a vision and a plan, but always be prepared for an opportunity.

Political stability and economic stability are key factors in people's hope for their country's future and their own.

CHAPTER 8

The "Charter" and Global Health Ethics

The importance of ethical considerations and engagement in global health is not a new idea. Taylor articulated basic principles in a paper published in 1966 and proposed a "Hippocratic Oath for Global Health" (see table).

Carl Taylor's Hippocratic Oath for Global Health
I will share the science and art by precept, by demonstration, and by every mode of teaching with other physicians regardless of their national origin.
I will try to help secure for the physicians in each country the esteem of their own people, and through collaborative work see that they get full credit.
I will strive to eliminate sources of disease everywhere in the world and not merely set up barriers to the spread of disease to my own people.
I will work for understanding of the diverse causes of diseases, including social, economic, and environmental.
I will promote the well-being of mankind in all its aspects, not merely the bodily, with sympathy and consideration for a people's culture and beliefs.
I will strive to prevent painful and untimely death, and also help parents to achieve a family size conforming to their desires and to their ability to care for their children.
In my concern with whole communities, I will never forget the needs of its individual members.

(Taylor, 1966).

Shortly after I returned to Michigan in 1993, the University of Michigan received a grant from the Gates Foundation called CHARTER, which stood for Collaborative Health Alliance for Reshaping Training, Education, and Research. This project had four objectives. The first was the creation of a document to guide the collaboration using a plan that described a process, and from the beginning we called this document "A Charter for Collaboration." Objective two was focused on strategies to improve data-driven policymaking objectives, including work by Margaret Kruk around medical student career decision making (Kruk et al., 2010). Objective three focused on enhancing transnational, inter-disciplinary, and interprofessional collaboration. Objective four sought to increase capacity building for research in Ghana (Anderson et al., 2014). The Charter for Collaboration was to establish the principle and guiding course of the program's technical work and create an ongo-ing and reflective process for providers. It grew into much more. We ended up with an excellent document that has been used as a model and template by other institutions and countries, allowing them to not have to recreate the process we had gone through and move directly to talking about and creating meaningful collaboration. The key guiding principles of the Charter were trust, mutual respect, communication, accountability, transparency, leadership, and sustainability. (A copy of the Charter is part of Appendix 1.)

The process for developing the Charter included a large number of Ghanaians from across numerous disciplines representing the univer-sities, the Ministry of Health, and a variety of Americans, including nurses, physicians, and advocates who, importantly, met at an out-of-the-way resort hotel overlooking Elmina Castle near Cape Coast (a remarkable former slave castle that famously brought tears to the eyes of President Barack Obama on his first visit to West Africa). The iso-lated location, with poor phone and internet connectivity and great conference and breakout areas, allowed the participants to focus on shared work over several productive days. The group formulated the Charter for Collaboration, which was signed in an impressive cere-mony, with copies of the signed Charter now hanging in Ann Arbor, the Ghana Ministry of Health, and the universities in Ghana.

The Charter process brought together many disparate existing collaborative agreements, MOUs (memoranda of understanding), and similar documents that had been the basis for international collaborations and global health partnership previously. In addition, the group consulted the specific language of previous documents including the Magna Carta, the Ghanaian Constitution, the US Declaration of Independence and Constitution, and the UN Universal Declaration of Human Rights. In addition, several members of the group brought expertise in feminist theory and feminist practice to the process and the discussion.

Once again documenting all this in a manuscript, both the process and the outcome were an important part of the project, and this is well described in the subsequent publication. It was thought it was very important to document not just the outcomes but the process, so that whatever part of the process, whether it was good or bad, could be reflected in subsequent approaches to global health collaboration and collaborative agreements and work.

The Elmina Declaration on Partnerships to Address Human Resources for Health from the Ghana-Michigan Collaborative Health Alliance Reshaping Training, Education, and Research, 2009

Preamble: This document is a Charter for Collaboration which describes the partnership between groups working in Michigan, USA and Ghana to improve human resources for health funded by the Bill and Melinda Gates Foundation

II. Conscious of the need to

1 Share experiences in medical education, research, innovative technology, and leadership among all partners
2. Develop and share technological and other educational resources efficiently and effectively
3. Develop resources to optimize and fully utilize education, training, and deployment of HRH
4. Improve the infrastructure for electronic communication, skills training, and clinical care

5. Expand the scope of research and translate research results into policy and educational initiatives

6. Recognize, identify, and involve appropriate HRH workers in the process

7. Expand and decentralize education and training into peripheral health facilities, district, public, and private

8. Develop a national government research infrastructure to fund national health research

9. Articulate principles that guide partnerships to lead to sustainable, mutually beneficial collaboration, namely:

TRUST MUTUAL RESPECT COMMUNICATION

ACCOUNTABILITY TRANSPARENCY LEADERSHIP

SUSTAINABILITY

Using the Ghana Charter and the background outlined in depth in the descriptive publication (Anderson, 2014), Ethiopia (see Chapter 10) adopted a very similar charter for collaboration document at the initiation of that program, with only appropriate and minor modifications for the Ethiopian context and cultures. In many ways the Charter has provided an important and readymade ethical framework and basis for that program.

There are several telling stories that exemplify some of the global health equity issues associated with well-meaning attempts by institutions and organizations of the Global North to engage in global health work. The tale of magnesium sulfate ($MgSO_4$) is one that exemplifies issues of supply chain and infrastructure, research ethics, and social justice. $MgSO_4$, sold commercially and manufactured cheaply as Epsom salts, is used medicinally by injection and intravenous infusion to prevent seizures and complications caused by preeclampsia, a common obstetric hypertensive disease of unknown cause. $MgSO_4$ has been commonly used in the United States to treat preeclampsia since its popularization by Doctor Nicholson J. Eastman of Johns Hopkins after research he had performed in Beijing, China, at Peking Union Medical College in the 1930s—research that he would have been unlikely to have been able to carry out in the United States because of the relative rarity of the disease and lack of enthusiasm at the time, by doctors and patients, for clinical research. Just as today, doctors traveled outside the United States to do research on diseases that were more common or in larger patient populations (like China) than existed in the United States. Interestingly, as we have heard, it was the selfsame Eastman who, during a UK-sponsored trip to Baltimore, had inspired a just-graduated British obstetrician/gynecologist, John Lawson, to pursue an international career, much later to join the External Advisory Board of the GPTP representing RCOG (see Chapter 3). Commonly used in the United States since the 1950s and 1960s, $MgSO_4$ was less commonly used, and often ridiculed, by western European practitioners and other international physicians, who often used other sedative and antiepileptic therapies to treat and manage the disease. To prove its value, an international, multicenter randomized clinical trial was initiated in July 1998 and conducted by a research unit in Oxford, United Kingdom, to determine the drug's therapeutic value. The obstetric unit at KATH in Kumasi, and its medical school OBGYN faculty led by department chair Doctor Kwabena Danso (remember him? the first graduate from the GPTP in Kumasi), was a participating center in the so-called MAGPIE (MAGnesium Sulphate for Prevention of Eclampsia) trial (Altman et al., 2002).

To complete the trial, $MgSO_4$, which was not clinically available in Ghana and certainly not part of the MOH list of recommended pharmaceuticals, was made available and paid for by the study team. It was, however, manufactured at several factories in Ghana as a nonmedical Epsom salt, as it was almost everywhere else in the world. The MAGPIE study concluded in November 2001, and its advantages and benefits over other therapy was reported in the *Lancet* in 2002 (Altman et al., 2002). $MgSO_4$ was now clearly the drug of choice, the standard of practice, for management of preeclampsia and eclampsia and the "gold standard" everywhere in the world. But the cessation of the MAGPIE trial in Kumasi led to the cessation of the availability of $MgSO_4$ at KATH, and its continued unavailability at every hospital in Ghana. The drug, while cheap and producible in a country where Epsom salts were used as a remedy for sore, aching feet, was not available in pharmaceutical grade. It took from 2002 to 2015 for the drug to appear on the national drug formulary and become widely available to hospitals for treatment of preeclampsia. Research had been done in Ghana, results that were immediately adopted in high-income countries across the world were produced, and yet, when the study was completed, the drug was completely unavailable in Ghana. Research ethics from this and other similar experiences now require attention to the design of new research and results implementation for those doing studies in LMIC, where the prevalence of the disease often makes recruitment and enrollment in studies easy and fast. New international clinical research guidelines and rules increasingly require—or should require—that studies proving efficacy in LMIC include a provision in their study design and implementation plan to make the drug immediately available in that country, to its people, for their benefit, if the drug's benefit is proven in the trial (Spector-Bagdady & Johnson, 2021).

Much of the most recent wave of enthusiasm for global health has been led by infectious disease internists and others expert in immunizations and epidemics. This has been in response to new outbreaks like Ebola and, especially, the resultant huge federal expenditures on prevention and mitigation projects funded by the President's Emergency Plan for AIDS Relief (PEPFAR), USAID, and the Centers for Disease Control and Prevention (CDC). These have been financial windfalls for infectious disease–focused projects in Africa and around the world and for the proliferation of university centers for global health in US universities. With a drawdown in PEPFAR and other funding, the interest in global health is waning in some of these academic institutions. Many of these problems are based on the real public-health fear of the introduction of HIV, Ebola, COVID-19, and other pathogens to the US from abroad. One critique of these pandemic/infectious disease–centric global health programs is their failure to develop long-term, sustainable, primary care infrastructure in the countries where they operate. An epidemiologic focus could narrowly pursue identification, containment, and mitigation, but ideally immunization, as a way to stop local or global spread of a disease. HIV programs have shown that when faced with a treatable but not curable infectious disease, long-term capacity to provide suppressive medication and provide chronic disease management is required. Health capacity, and to some degree human resource capacity, is required for the long term.

As an obstetrician, I recognize this sustainable primary care as requisite for dealing with issues of maternal and child health, especially the maternal component. Major inroads were made on reducing childhood mortality with the worldwide introduction of immunizations to prevent deaths from childhood infections (measles, mumps, tetanus, diphtheria), and oral rehydration therapy reduced infant mortality from diarrheal diseases. However, as Rosenfield pointed out in "Where is the M in MCH?" (A. Rosenfield & Maine, 1985), the common causes of maternal mortality require the availability of a trained health professional. There are no immunizations for postpartum hemorrhage, hypertensive disease of pregnancy, or puerperal sepsis. Maternal health and the increasing worldwide burden of noncommunicable diseases (diabetes, high blood pressure, etc.) require sustained health service availability and capacity. The epidemiologic model of early testing, case identification, quarantine, containment, and vaccination simply will not work.

A case example is Salome Karwah, who was on the cover of *Time* magazine as a 2014 "Person of the Year" Ebola fighter. She survived the Ebola that killed her physician father and nurse mother and much of her family on the health compound where they worked. She survived Ebola because of the expensive ICU care she received from the Ebola medical teams created at the nexus of the Ebola pandemic in her native Liberia. As a rare survivor, she committed herself to help in the care of other Ebola victims. She was an example of a supreme victory of massive financial and resource commitment in West Africa to treat and prevent the spread of a terrible epidemic. This expenditure undoubtedly prevented the much-feared spread of Ebola further across West Africa and to the shores of Europe and America. After the epidemic was quelched through modern epidemiologic and medical means, the Ebola teams left Liberia and the neighboring involved countries. One year later, after giving birth to a fourth child, Salome suddenly developed postpartum eclampsia and died on her family compound. Hers was probably a preventable death if only her high blood pressure had been identified and treated with $MgSO_4$, and more importantly, if $MgSO_4$ and antihypertensive therapies had even been available at the health center where she became ill and had seizures (Spector-Bagdady & Johnson, 2021). It also would have helped if caregivers, afraid that she had recurrent Ebola, had been trained and prepared to care for her complications of pregnancy. This is another example where global health ethics requires an in-depth understanding of global health disparities and inequities, and attention to social justice and income inequality, especially between the Global North and the Global South.

The mindset of many epidemiologic infectious disease initiatives, and that of European orthopedic surgeons who, as we shall see (Chapter 9), tried to export their Eurocentric model of trauma services to Ghana when no ambulance or emergency services even existed, are both examples of a failure to think about sustained primary care capacity building. Primary care public health systems and resources are necessary for sustained public health and advanced health care systems to develop in LMIC. Treating HIV long term with ART [antiretroviral therapy] medication requires an ongoing supply chain and a system that can deliver therapy to those infected. This was an important lesson from the successes of PEPFAR. Epidemic management does not provide on-the-ground capacity for sustained, long-term health care or management of noninfectious chronic disease. Preventive and chronic HIV services offer an example of continuity of care that requires sustainability.

The Ghana Project developed sustainable public health capacity and infrastructure for primary care (Anderson, 2019), just as we will see that an emergency medicine training program will provide sustainable services at the Accident and Emergency Centre at KATH-KNUST (Chapter 9).

As Parikh has pointed out, global health ethics presents substantial issues not usually considered to be of primary importance in clinical health ethics (Parikh, 2010). The four pillars of classic Western clinical ethics are (in order): nonmaleficence (captured in the dictum "*primo non nocere*," or "first, do no harm"); beneficence (doing the right thing and doing good for the patient); patient autonomy; and social justice (including equity in accessibility, affordability, availability, acceptability, and accountability). It has become increasingly clear since the rapid increase in interest and involvement of medical schools from high-income countries in global health that these clinical pillars are important but inadequate in appropriate transnational and transcultural partnership (Anderson et al., 2017; Kekulawala & Johnson 2018; Nordling, 2017; Spector-Bagdady & Johnson, 2021; Shah & Wu, 2008; Wall, 2012). These are required, but not enough; global health is about more than "first, do no harm." Of course, all clinical interactions anywhere in the world must avoid causing harm and must provide care that is in the best interest of a patient who is giving truly informed consent. The lessons of Nuremberg, the Tuskegee and Guatemala syphilis experiments, and the Belmont Report have all made it clear that the patient's autonomy and rights as a clinical and research subject must be respected. But global health programs require attention to other detailed collaborative principles that are well covered and summed up in the details of the Charter document—principles that ultimately guide partnerships that lead to sustainable, mutually beneficial collaboration: trust, mutual respect, communication, accountability, transparency, leadership, and sustainability.

Lessons Learned

Key principles to guide global health initiatives are trust, mutual respect, communication, accountability, transparency, leadership, and sustainability.

Global health partnership relationships and rules are best articulated and agreed upon prospectively.

The Charter model can serve as a template for ethical academic global health collaborations.

CHAPTER 9

"Sometimes They Just Walk in Your Door": Other Disciplines and Schools

Emergency Medicine at KATH

One successor of the postgraduate obstetrics and gynecology training program in Ghana has been the emergency medicine program at KATH in Kumasi. That, too, has its story. During a visit to KATH, I was asked by my Ghanaian hosts if I would like to see the early construction of the new Accident and Emergency Centre (Emergency Department). There was just a hole in the ground and some basic cement outlines of a large building, but it all looked like it had the potential to be very modern, with a large space for trauma bays and large emergency intake rooms. When I asked how emergency services were going to be provided, I was told that the Departments of Medicine and Surgery were going to share the space and provide consultation. By the 1990s, I knew that was not the model for contemporary emergency medicine. As a medical student and resident, I had trained in county and university hospitals, where "medicine" and "surgery" split duties. Coverage was usually by interns and internal medicine residents with staffing by experienced nurses: patients were triaged (sorted by acuity, usually by intake nurses or even sometimes a desk clerk) to medicine and surgery, female and male. Trauma, obvious surgical cases (fractures, wounds), and hemo-dynamically unstable patients were prioritized, and most others had to wait for an evaluation. Everything and anything, from dying nursing home patients, to colds, flu, and drug overdoses came in, often inef-ficiently using emergency services for routine, basic health care. This was, of course, compounded by uninsured or under-insured patients who had nowhere else to go for care.

By the mid-1970s, a new specialty, emergency medicine, was devel-oping in such US centers as the University of Cincinnati. I was lucky to practice with a team of mostly Cincinnati-trained "emergency medicine" doctors at Andrews Air Force Base from 1983 to 1985. These emergency medicine physicians specialized in resuscitation, triage, and evaluation. They quickly sorted patients and got them seen as needed by consultants, such as OBGYNs like me. They ordered the appropri-ate laboratory tests and imaging (x-rays, CT scans, ultrasounds), and the patients were often "worked up" with a clear diagnosis and ready, if needed, for admission or surgery by the time I got to the Emergency Department. I had also previously seen the "shock trauma" model developed by the visionary Doctor R. Adams Cowley at the University of Maryland, across town from my fellowship at Johns Hopkins, and I was sold on that too. (The Shock Trauma Center is the designated destination for the president of the United States if he is ever severely injured in the Washington, DC, area. Ronald Reagan should have been transported there when he was shot, but the severity of his gunshot wounds was not immediately or appropriately appreciated, and he went to a local DC hospital, where his trauma care was delayed.) This model recognized the developing concept of the "golden hour" that had been learned on the recent battlefields of Vietnam, where major casualty victims who were rapidly resuscitated and stabilized with the first sixty minutes had the best chances of intact survival. Johns Hopkins Hospital still used the old medicine/surgery model, and after my return there from the military in 1985, I was on a committee that recommended the establishment of a Department of Emergency Medicine and a residency program, but this recommendation was not accepted by the powerful Departments of Medicine and Surgery. Their leaders knew the Emergency Department was a major source of admissions to the hospital and economically important, therefore administrative control was desirable to maintain control of the flow of patients.

One other prior experience also influenced my thinking at the time. When I received my honorary fellowship at the West African College of Surgeons at its 2003 annual meeting in Abuja, Nigeria, the conference theme was "Trauma Care in West Africa." There were presentations by several German orthopedic trauma surgeons of the "European" model (I think it was a mostly German model), in which trauma care was organized and managed around accidents and motor vehicle trauma. Orthopedic surgeons and trauma surgeons flew in helicopters with field resuscitation capacity to pick up trauma victims on the Autobahn or the site of their trauma, where they were resuscitated, stabilized, and transported back to the closest major trauma/reanimation center for management. The presenters described a meticulously organized system for rapid communications and notification, deployment of their well-equipped helicopters, orthopedic/trauma surgeon–centric stabilization, and finally, transport back to fully equipped trauma centers. I thought this airborne trauma surgeon–dependent model was not feasible; it was not even imaginable in West Africa. Ghana lacked good roads, helicopters, an organized ambulance service, and an organized communication network. I thought, rather, that an emergency medicine physician–centric model—where emergency medicine–trained physicians saw the patients who were brought to them, managed their stabilization and evaluation, and triaged the patients to an appropriate specialty/subspecialty for admission or surgery—was what West Africa needed if the opportunity ever arose to enhance emergency care. In 2003 this did not seem likely anytime soon.

All this to say that my immediate response a few years later to the construction of a new accident and emergency (A&E) center at KATH was to think that here in Kumasi was an opportunity to introduce a new specialty, a new way of caring for patients, and a new administrative mindset at a Ghanaian academic medical center and do it in a newly constructed space designed specifically so that the new functionality could fill an appropriate new space. After all, function often follows form, and form can serve to change practice, behavior, and culture. New physical structures can disrupt organizational and behavioral structures. The time was right for emergency medicine at KATH. The planned building design could change to accommodate this new emergency medicine model and abandon the old "medical/surgical" model. Functionality would also be enhanced by the planned introduction of a new electronic medical record system in the Accident and Emergency Centre. But the building was beginning to go up and I had to move quickly.

I met the same day with hospital leadership at KATH and, within days in Accra, with the rector of the GCPS, Professor Paul Nyame, to propose the new clinical care paradigm and an associated training program. The GCPS would be the "home" of any new postgraduate training program, so their buy-in was important. As luck would have it, Professor Nyame, who had previously visited Michigan in conjunction with the GPTP exchanges, had, early in his career as an internist, directed the Accident and Emergency Centre at KBTH and knew there had to be a better way. He immediately grasped the merit of this new specialty of "emergency medicine." Everyone I spoke with was interested and supportive of the concept. I was a trusted and respected agent in Ghana, and the timing was perfect. Immediately upon my return to Ann Arbor I picked up the phone (I had become more comfortable doing that) and called the chair of the newly formed Department of Emergency Medicine at the University of Michigan, Doctor Bill Barsan. Yes, even Michigan was a relatively late adopter of emergency medicine, its acceptance blocked, unsurprisingly, by the Departments of Medicine and Surgery. Doctor Barsan was a board-certified emergency medicine physician and, when I first met him, chief of the Division of Emergency Medicine in the Department of Surgery. He became the inaugural chair of the department when emergency medicine became its own program. Doctor Barsan and I had worked on a number of projects before, respected each other, and he had heard me talk about our OBGYN Ghana partnership. "Yes!" was the answer to my phone call. Bill was interested in considering a global emergency medicine initiative by his department. He immediately identified a Ghanaian-born, Cincinnati-trained emergency medicine junior faculty member, Doctor Rockefeller Oteng, and a core of other interested faculty colleagues. Together they developed a proposal and funded an exploratory trip to Ghana, where plans for an emergency medicine training program at KATH, supported by the Emergency Medicine Department at UM, were made. Further funding from the Fogarty International Center, the National Institutes of Health (NIH), and professional societies followed. I think the reputation of the GPTP and the strong, established, and well-known partnership with Michigan helped in building an early trust relationship around the emergency medicine program. This would be a first for West Africa.

As Doctor Oteng and his colleagues thought carefully about how to develop this emergency medicine training, they involved not only KATH and its administration that was building the new Accident and Emergency Centre but also the KNUST School of Medical Sciences and the Ghana College of Physicians and Surgeons. The Ghana College was interested in supporting the establishment of the specialty and developed an entirely novel curriculum so that emergency medicine physicians could be trained and receive GCPS certification and fellowship in Ghana.

Doctors Barsan and Oteng, from their very first trip to Kumasi, assisted in revising the building plans for the new A&E center. Before it opened, they arranged for Ghanaian critical care nurses to come to UM to observe, share protocols and policies, and "learn to be emergency medicine nurses" before their return to KATH. This nursing exchange was very beneficial to the establishment of the emergency medicine services and the department in Kumasi, and the nurses, as they always do, unquestionably played an important role in training the first Ghanaian emergency medicine postgraduates. When it opened, Michigan emergency medicine faculty and a Ghana-born UK "accident room" specialist doctor were there working side-by-side with Ghanaian specialist doctors. The first emergency medicine residents started at KATH in 2009 and finished in 2012, and subsequently, emergency medicine physicians trained at KATH have populated not only its own emergency department but emergency departments in private hospitals around the region (Martel et al., 2014; Osei-Ampofo et al., 2013, 2018; Oteng & Donkor, 2014; Oteng et al., 2020; Rominski et al., 2015).

As an important part of the preparation for the opening of the A&E center, Doctor Oteng and his colleagues worked to advance organization of the Ghana National Ambulance Service to provide rapid pickup, assessment, and transport of accident and emergency victims. A radio-link communication system was established so the emergency medicine physician and A&E nurses could communicate with the Ghana National Ambulance Service (just like on TV and at the University of Maryland Shock Trauma center in Baltimore, which established "SYSCOM" (I still love to say that word) to communicate with the Maryland State Police helicopter system, which would then fly out to pick up trauma patients from the highway or other accident site. I knew it well because, as a maternal-fetal medicine fellow, I regularly used the system to communicate—get it?—to arrange helicopter transport of sick, high-risk pregnant patients for care at Hopkins. My training and experience had prepared me for the concept of triage and transfer of high-risk patients—whether from a train wreck or an unanticipated pregnancy complication on the rural eastern shore of Maryland. My experience and training, no doubt, prepared me to identify this once-in-a-lifetime opportunity at KATH. **But for** that trip through the dirty and dusty construction site of the future A&E center, I am convinced this successful program never would have happened when it did. The emergency medicine program continues to thrive with frequent trips by Doctor Oteng and his colleagues to Ghana and visits to Michigan for Ghanaian trainees. A fellowship in critical care emergency medicine has been started at KATH, led by Doctor Oteng, and his many publications have described the development of the program and now describe its continuing accomplishments and research contributions (Martel et al., 2014; Osei-Ampofo et al., 2013; Oteng et al., 2014, 2019; Rominski et al., 2015). These scholarly publications have served to advance the academic careers of

Doctor Oteng and the Ghanaian emergency medicine faculty that he has helped train and mentored. KBTH has recently provided financial support for some of its own doctors as emergency medicine trainees at KATH, with the expectation that they will return to Accra and help move KBTH's antiquated medicine/surgery model into the twenty-first century and extend the "emergency medicine" model further across the country.

The importance of building the right space for the desired function became something that I was very sensitized to and aware of after this experience. When we started in 2000 at Michigan to plan the construction of the new Von Voigtlander Women's Hospital, we were very intentional in the process. We spent more years planning then we ended up spending in the construction phase. (That was quite probably related.) As part of the design process, we asked ourselves how we thought we wanted to practice in 2040 and how we could build a hospital that would allow us to do that in 2010. We built a hospital that allowed us to move entirely to an electronic record on the day we moved into the hospital. We also changed our nursing and physician models of care at the time of the move to the new hospital. I learned from the experience in Ghana that the idea of first thinking intensively about how we intended to practice medicine in the space and about the functionality of the space should drive our design considerations. In this model, function ultimately follows, and is often driven by, a carefully determined form. This approach also helped us on several occasions when we wanted to change our practice—for example, to provide one uniform type of nursing for all maternity patients. This change was daunting and difficult, but we found that by changing our space configuration and parameters, the resultant change to the desired functionality was sometimes not as difficult, and sometimes "it just happens" because of how the new space is used (actually, how it was planned). This is yet another example of global health experiences and lessons having substantial "domestic" benefits and applicability. Innumerable lessons that I learned in sub-Saharan Africa have applied to the work that I do in the United States. People always say "I always get more than I put in" to global work, and it is true.

Midwifery

It was identified early on that success in resident education would require the support of nursing graduate education, and nursing was a requisite discipline for any OBGYN or MCH initiative to be successful. Jody Lori, CNM, PhD, and Carol Boyd, RN, PhD, activated a certified nurse midwife (CNM) faculty training program, and Professor Lori, who had extensive experience in Liberia, began networking with Ghanaian midwives and nurses and eventually got a training grant to support capacity building in Ghana. They were very involved in the Charter formation at Elmira and were an excellent way, through our strong, collegial, collaborative, and friendly relationship, to role-model and mentor interprofessional education (Dzomeku et al., 2017, 2022; Rominski et al., 2017).

Breast Surgery at KATH: Lisa Newman, MD, MPH

Sometimes opportunities are identified in the field, such as the GPTP that began after a trip to Ghana and went on to become the first piece of the "Platform" that is the UM-Ghana partnership. Sometimes they are identified on the ground, like the emergency medicine residency program that arose, along with the accident and emergency center that inspired it. Sometimes the opportunity just knocks on your office door. Such was the case for Doctor Lisa Newman.

Lisa Newman, MD, MPH, was a young, clinically astute and aspiring academic breast surgeon in the Department of Surgery at UM. She was also trained in public health and was particularly interested in the epidemiology of breast cancer, specifically the racial disparities in diagnosis and outcome in the United States, where black women present with later-stage, more advanced disease and die younger and at a higher rate than white women. Doctor Newman had established a robust subspecialty surgical practice caring for breast cancer patients. She was highly regarded by colleagues for the outstanding surgical care and empathy she provided. But like any young academic, she had yet to establish her own strong academic research niche. While interested in health disparities and in racial inequities in care and outcome, she did not yet have a short and clear "elevator speech" to quickly summarize her research and publications to date and describe her desired career trajectory. She came to my office, quiet and petite because that is her style, but also, no doubt, because of her conditioning in the patriarchal hierarchies of surgery. She wondered if there were opportunities to extend her epidemiologic research to women with breast cancer to Ghana (Trimble & Helzlsouer, 2016). Were there ever!

I thought that the Kumasi surgery department would be most receptive to a US collaborator. I knew there was a designated "oncology center" in the planning and early building phase at that point, and there were basic radiation oncology treatment machines and a recently returned Ghanaian radiation oncologist well trained in the West. A few introductions were made to surgical department leaders at KNUST through my OBGYN department friends, and Doctor Newman was off for an exploratory visit. Her success over more than a decade has recently been described in a scholarly publication (Jiagge et al., 2016) authored by the many, people who assisted, worked with, and benefited from Doctor Newman's engaged academic global health work in Ghana.

Her achievements include a breast care clinic at KATH and Ghana-UM virtual video interdisciplinary breast cancer care conferences that include breast pathologists, medical oncologists, radiation oncologists, surgical oncologists, and many, many trainees. Teleconferencing is available for consultation with breast cancer pathology experts on problem cases. Doctor Newman developed a team that made possible the transportation of breast tumor specimens to UM from KATH for pathologic evaluation and genetics research. In her laboratory, Doctor Newman was able to demonstrate a high prevalence of poor-prognosis triple-negative (estrogen receptor–negative, progesterone receptor–negative, HER2 /neu–negative) breast cancer in Ghanaian women. This led to a major breakthrough, beginning with the recognition of the high prevalence of triple-negative breast cancer (TNBC) across Ghana. TNBC is fairly rare in American white women and intermediate in African American women. Many African American women are descendants of West African slaves from Ghana and the surrounding region (Nigeria, Sierra Leone, Cote d'Ivoire, Benin), where their ancestors were sold by rival tribes into slavery and taken across the Middle Passage. Perhaps there was a relationship between African American women and their West African female ancestors in their genetic patterns of breast cancer. This important groundbreaking discovery by Doctor Newman, only possible because she worked in Ghana, started a clinic, and did research on the patients she cared for suggests that there is a major genetic factor that causes aggressive disease and high mortality in African American women and therefore suggests approaches to prevention. Equally important, this finding in Ghana will be used to inform how breast care programs are organized for prevention, early detection, and early evidence-based care—which for Ghanaians may even be personalized, that is, directed specifically at TNBC. Further work by Doctor Newman, now professor of surgery and founding medical director for the International Center for the Study of Breast Cancer Subtypes at Cornell Medical Center in New York City, has shown that in parts of East Africa, TNBC is much less common, suggesting that careful genetic studies will be necessary across Africa to identify differences in the types, prognoses, and treatments of breast cancer.

Doctor Newman's scholarship and numerous publications have resulted in not only rapid promotion to professor but also national and international attention. Doctor Evelyn Jiagge, a Ghanaian breast surgeon, has completed a PhD in breast cancer basic science at the University of Michigan under the tutelage of Doctor Newman. After a postdoctoral fellowship, it is anticipated she will return to Ghana and provide clinical care in the KATH breast center, continue her basic science research, and become an academic superstar and woman leader, like her mentor.

Doctor Newman was attentive to and followed the lessons of the GPTP and the "Michigan Model" and adapted them with strong input from colleagues, collaborators, and friends she developed in Ghana. She has established a model international center that is worthy and capable of replication and modification for other sustained academic partnerships. Doctor Newman has shown how important basic science and translational research can lead to new insights into a common disease like breast cancer; that building clinic and laboratory research capacity on the ground is possible and necessary to be successful in low-income countries; and once again, that sustained academic partnerships can lead to long-standing gains in clinical care, education, research, and capacity building (Jiagge et al., 2016).

Global Health Design and Engineering: Kathleen Sienko

Another person who "showed up" in my office was Kathleen Sienko, a Harvard-MIT- trained biomedical engineer and UM College of Engineering assistant professor. (The Harvard-MIT biomedical engineering graduate program is probably unique in that it engages the engineering graduate students in the preclinical science years of medical school at Harvard Medical School before completing engineering PhD at MIT. I suspect this strongly encourages future interdisciplinary and interprofessional skills and abilities.) She was interested in global health and global engineering, especially for undergraduate students. She was specifically teaching mechanical engineering undergraduates but had also worked with interdisciplinary teams of undergraduate students, including those from other schools and colleges (Nursing, Public Health, and the College of Literature, Science, and the Arts, or LS&A).

Kumasi was the perfect space to send her teams to, and she joined them there for end-user assessment as a regular part of the design science and engineering process that I came to admire and respect. Her teams came to the UM Birth Center to watch nurses and doctors in action and to observe deliveries and Cesarean deliveries before going to Ghana. There, they worked on identifying projects of local interest—again, note the respect and attention to end user from the onset. Then, the students returned to UM, did their design project, and returned to present the "product" to the end users in country.

Kathleen developed close links with the School of Engineering at KNUST and the Department of Biomedical Engineering faculty and students in Accra. Undergraduate and graduate engineering students worked with undergraduate LS&A students, School of Nursing students, and medical students with different mixes in different years as an excellent example of interprofessional health education (IPE).

Kathleen Sienko has been recognized with promotion to professor, tenure, and selection as a prestigious Thurnau Professor. She cofounded the UM Center for Socially Engaged Design (C-SED), and she now directs the College of Engineering's Global Health Design Initiative (GHDI). She has created and implemented curricular and cocurricular experiential design offerings through GHDI, which aims to train a new generation of engineers and, more broadly, designers to communicate and collaborate with stakeholders to identify and define needs and develop and implement solutions to address essential health care challenges. She and her colleagues have done work in Ghana to design and build birth tables (Hessburg et al., 2012; Perosky et al., 2012) and obstetric simulation devices (Andreatta et al., 2012), and in Uganda to build an adult male circumcision device for use in programs to reduce the transmission of HIV (Lemmermen et al., 2010). She has also played a major role in developing the exciting discipline of global health design (Mohedas et al., 2014, 2015; Sienko et al., 2013, 2014, 2018; Sabet Sarvestani & Sienko, 2014; Winget et al., 2015).

Interview with Professor Kathleen Sienko

Professor Kathleen Sienko is now an Arthur F. Thurnau Professor, professor of mechanical engineering, professor of biomedical engineering, and Miller Faculty Scholar in the College of Engineering at the University of Michigan. She also directs the Laboratory for Innovation in Global Health Technology (LIGHT). She received a BS in Materials Engineering at the University of Kentucky, an SM in Aeronautics and Astronautics from MIT, and a PhD in Medical Engineering and Bioastronautics from the Harvard-MIT Division of Health Sciences and Technology. Her research and pedagogical interests include rehabilitation engineering, biomechanics, medical device design, design for resource-constrained settings, and design science. I interviewed her about her global health trajectory and her programs in Ghana:

T (Tim Johnson) Talk a little bit about your personal journey. I know you started off interested in astronautics and space travel with NASA as a goal; you did your engineering degree at Kentucky and then moved to the biomedical PhD combined program at MIT and Harvard. When did global health get on your personal radar screen?

K (Kathleen Sienko) As a PhD student.

T So you were already past engineering into a PhD program.

K Yes. Since elementary school, I aspired to be an astronaut and pursued degrees that would support me in achieving that goal. During my master's research at MIT, I began studying human physiological changes to microgravity and worked on developing interventions for long-duration space flight, such as a short-radius centrifuge for a manned mission to Mars. Around the time of the space shuttle Columbia disaster, it seemed unlikely that the US space program would relax their eligibility criteria for the astronaut corps specifically their vision criterion. As a fifth grader, I tore the retina in my left eye during a sports accident, so it didn't seem possible to continue pursuing that dream.

    I started to look into other career options; I did some soul-searching, took some time off from the PhD program, and enrolled in a few science and technology policy and international studies night classes while working as a research engineer. Despite an interest in science and technology policy, I followed the advice of mentors and decided to stick with engineering versus switching to a policy-based doctoral degree, with the idea that down the road, I'd be able to transition to policy-related work.

    When I returned to the PhD program, I joined a lab that was doing space research. But they were working with people who had vestibular deficits as analogs to astronauts who had been in space for an extended period of time. For example, people with compensated vestibulopathies can have similar balance-related symptoms and challenges to astronauts returning from extended stays on the International Space Station.

    My research focused on developing tests that could detect subtle balance deficits and balance aids for this earth-based population.

Those research projects initiated the shift in my focus to an earth-based population and afforded me the opportunity to apply my engineering background to solve problems with the potential for achieving short-term impact.

T I like the term "earth-based population."

K The clinical preceptorship component of my PhD program further increased my interest in applying engineering to solve earth-based medical challenges and introduced me to the field of global health. I was assigned the West Roxbury VA Hospital for my first two preceptorships, and we had an option of completing a third clinical preceptorship or conducting a short-term research project in a laboratory outside of our primary research area. Around the time that I was trying to make the decision to either complete a third preceptorship or find a different lab to rotate through, I attended a required seminar series and heard Doctor Kristian Olson from Massachusetts General Hospital speak about his experiences practicing medicine in a refugee camp. I became very excited about the prospect of completing my third preceptorship at an international field site and specifically in a resource-constrained setting, but my program turned down my request to complete my preceptorship at a refugee camp for safety reasons. However, they connected me with Doctor Shiladitya Sengupta, who helped me to set up an opportunity to obtain a related experience in India at the All-India Institute of Medical Sciences (AIIMS).

My experiences at AIIMS, as well as municipal and private hospitals within the New Delhi area, turned out to be career-changing experiences—I saw completely different constraints with respect to the provision of health care and the use of health care technologies. Specifically, I saw the lack of technology that was appropriately designed to meet local Indian needs, and I saw the misuse of technology that was designed for use in high-income country settings; for example, catheters that were meant to be disposable were sterilized and reused up to five times to reduce the cost to patients. There were also a few examples of novel medical devices that were under development by American universities to address local Indian needs that did not take into consideration broader contextual constraints such as cultural and social constraints.

So when I interviewed for a faculty position at Michigan, I expressed my desire to develop educational opportunities comparable to my experiences in India for undergraduate students. I was fortunate to have had the opportunity to conduct clinical observations in a low-/middle-income country, but it was during the last summer of my PhD program, which is fairly late with respect to shaping career trajectories in academia.

T So you wanted to give students an opportunity earlier than you had.

K Yes. I wanted to give students an opportunity earlier in their academic careers. And I thought that it would be advantageous to have that type of an experience as an undergraduate because it would allow students to potentially pivot their early career path prior to taking their first job or continuing their education. It was a transformative experience for me, and I wanted others to have the opportunity for a similar experience.

When I arrived at Michigan, I tried to figure out who was doing what and where. I didn't have any initial luck finding faculty in the medical school that were doing work in India, which was an obvious starting point for me based on my experiences the previous year.

I eventually connected with Global REACH and Doctor Frank Anderson, an OBGYN who was performing research in Ghana and who got me to you. In parallel, I identified an opportunity through the UM Global Intercultural Experience for Undergraduates [GIEU] program to create a faculty-led experiential learning program at an international field site, and I approached Frank about the possibility of coleading a field site with me in Ghana focused on maternal health needs assessments.

We didn't read the fine print that said that as coleaders we both would have to spend five to six weeks at the field site. So when our GIEU proposal was accepted and Frank said he couldn't travel for that length of time, I decided to solely lead the student cohort. Due to a flight delay, I think I arrived in Ghana a couple days or maybe just one day before the eleven students arrived.

T   So what year was that?

K   This was 2008.

T   Okay.

K   The GIEU students selected for my field site were a mix of people transitioning between their freshman and sophomore, sophomore and junior, and junior and senior years.

T   And were some of them biomedical engineering students?

K   We had one engineering student out of the entire group of eleven. The other students were in Communication, Movement Science, African American Studies, Women's Studies, Psychology, English, Sociology, Anthropology, Neuroscience, and Nursing. Frank [Anderson] was pivotal in shaping the initial partnership, and he introduced me to clinical faculty at Komfo Anokye Teaching Hospital [KATH]. He also helped me to prepare the students and he met with them in Ghana during a visit he made there. All my contacts were established through the existing UM-Ghana platform. At the time, Doctor Kwabena Danso was department head of OBGYN at KATH. He welcomed us and hosted the students in his department for approximately five weeks while they performed observations and interviews for the purpose of identifying unmet maternal health needs.

T   So you used the same kind of engineering process that you had been trained with, right? That kind of needs identification.

K   I didn't have formal training in needs-finding. I tried to formalize the methods that I used in India to understand needs and shortcomings in existing health care technologies. I was learning as I was doing, and my experiences in India and through GIEU informed subsequent curricular development around the topics of needs assessment and design ethnography. After my experience in 2008, I decided to offer a second GIEU field site at KATH in 2009. I also had the chance to hire a former participant as a student field site coleader. I think you and I met around 2009 through Frank. You formally brought me into the UM-Ghana partnership and included me in some important meetings related to the development of the partnership. Your support opened numerous doors for me and facilitated numerous relationships with clinical faculty and trainees within your department. Our UM-based engineering-OBGYN collaboration has made a huge impact on the success of this work.

At the time, GIEU only allowed individual faculty to lead up to two field sites, so in 2010 (for the third cohort of students) I was on my own without GIEU's infrastructural support. However, I had the support of the extant MichiGhana platform, including Global REACH, and the KATH OBGYN leadership. During the initial experiences with GIEU, I began to identify needs that could potentially be pursued through the UM Mechanical Engineering capstone design class. However, during 2008 and 2009, the students that identified needs in Ghana were not the same students who developed concept solutions to address the needs within the capstone design course. In 2010, I gained that continuity by having the same students that identified needs in Ghana address those needs in the capstone design course. In 2010 I traveled with eleven students, approximately half of whom were engineering students. I also received permission for the non-engineering students to enroll in the mechanical engineering capstone design course.

In 2011 I piloted a program with Professor Elsie Effah Kaufmann from the Biomedical Engineering Department at the University of Ghana and Professor Samuel Obed from the OBGYN Department at the Korle Bu Teaching Hospital (KBTH). We also worked with Doctor Moses Musaazi from Makerere University in Uganda. This pilot program involved four engineering students conducting a needs assessment at KBTH—two from the University of Ghana, one from Makerere University, and one from the University of Michigan. From that point forward, I ran multiple field sites per year, expanding to China the following year, and eventually Ethiopia, Kenya, and now a domestic field site in Flint, MI. Our collaboration with the University of Ghana and KBTH has continued since 2011, and we typically match two to four UM students with two to four University of Ghana students. The group typically spends approximately six to eight weeks following a formal process to identify and define needs. The University of Ghana students design solutions to needs identified at KBTH during their two-semester biomedical engineering capstone design sequence, while the UM students plug into the single-semester UM mechanical engineering capstone design course.

T   Please explain how you developed the idea that on-the-ground needs assessment in low-income countries is useful. Is that part of the usual thinking of the mechanical engineering process and the design science process? How did that coalesce with you in thinking about how you were going to develop the process on the ground in Ghana?

K   My global health design educational programs were informed by my experiences in India; in particular, after seeing one example of a very well-intentioned design project that was undertaken by a renowned US institution. I don't think the US students or the faculty member that was leading that effort had a good understanding of the context of use of the technology.

They designed something that was functional, but it wasn't adopted because it was perceived by the end users to eliminate their jobs. Generally, the design team didn't take into consideration the local social and cultural constraints. Their focus seemed to be on addressing functional and economic constraints.

It became clear that you can't assume that there is a need unless you collect ground truth data and that you can't define the need by sitting in a lab or classroom at the University of Michigan. You have to codefine needs with stakeholders who are intimately familiar with the context of use. In terms of the process that I used, it wasn't entirely unique. In 2010, *Biodesign: The Process of Innovating Medical Technologies* by Zenios, Makower, and Yock was published, which mirrored the commonsense approaches that I had used in India in 2006 and had been using to teach my students since 2008. In general, I challenge my student teams to identify as many needs as they can—I ask them to identify at least one hundred unmet needs and refine them until they appropriately capture the real needs. Then we develop need prioritization rubrics—these are typically a series of coarse and fine filters to identify the highest priority and/or most appropriate needs. We work closely with key stakeholders, for example, the OBGYN leadership at KATH and KBTH, to make sure that we take into consideration factors that are important to them.

We also prioritize needs that would be appropriate for senior engineering students to pursue in their capstone design courses. It has taken quite a bit of time and experience to figure out which needs make the most sense to pursue. Ideally, I want to strike a balance between pursuing needs that have the potential for either short- or long-term impact. There are certain needs that are very difficult to address through a single-semester capstone design class, such as needs that are best addressed through complex electromechanical systems. Medical devices in general are challenging because of the regulatory approval processes. Other needs—for example, simulators or trainers—can be developed over a shorter period of time and, if shown to be effective, can be transferred to our clinical partners for use.

My current strategy is to diversify the portfolio of health technology projects that we pursue. With respect to medical devices, you're in it for the long game, especially if you're starting from the needs-finding stage and working within an academic setting. We can only take a global health technology so far within the academic setting, and then we need to start a company or find someone who wants to license it.

Over the years we've tried to carefully pick topics that students could tackle within a relatively short period of time to demonstrate initial proof of concept. We repeat the project if it looks like there's an opportunity to further develop the idea and potentially translate it beyond the classroom. If an idea has legs to stand on and if a student team isn't interested in creating a startup company, I seek competitive grant funding opportunities to hire graduate students to further develop the idea.

My experiences over the past ten years have shaped the way that I think about the science of design. There have been a lot of lessons learned through our work. There are shortcomings in the literature in terms of educational materials that provide adequate support for novice designers to learn how to be effective design ethnographers. I think there's good information out there about high-level approaches to doing design ethnography, but, for example, the nuanced methodological details needed to conduct an effective design interview to elicit product requirements are lacking.

We've learned a lot through the process of doing the design work ourselves, as well as through coaching students. Our own work has sprouted research thrusts in several areas including design ethnography learning trajectories, product requirements elicitation methodologies, prototype usage methodologies for stakeholder engagement, etc. For example, a rough prototype or sketch may be effective at the University of Michigan when engaging with a resident or an attending, but will that same type of prototype be equally effective when one is engaging with comparable stakeholder groups in Ghana? It's been interesting to see differences in the effectiveness of prototypes for communicating ideas with various stakeholder groups as the type of the prototype varies.

In general, our process yields a large number of needs and a large number of potential concept solutions. Whenever possible, we try to find resources to support the further development of the most promising concept solutions. There have been several needs that have transitioned beyond the classroom. One of the students from the 2010 cohort cofounded a company that has just completed clinical trials in Ethiopia for a blood salvage device. A cervical cancer screening simulator project from 2012 is in use in Ghana and is being further developed by the original two students that identified the need. We're also preparing to test an assistive contraceptive insertion device in a small clinical trial based on a need identified in Ethiopia in 2013 by two PhD students in my research group. In parallel, as we identify gaps within the design science and engineering education literature, we've applied for funding to conduct research to address those gaps.

In general, our students gain a tremendous amount of firsthand experience and education from these clinical immersion and design ethnography experiences. In many cases, it feels like a one-way street that disproportionately favors our students. It has been very important to me to think about how to equalize the playing field—can we give as much as we receive? One of the strategies that we've come up with in addition to diversifying our portfolio of global health technologies is to invest time and energy in developing partnerships with African universities, with an emphasis on engineering, in order to contribute to their capacity building efforts.

T   And can you talk a little bit about the importance of that kind of, that bilateral engagement?

K   Yes, it's been a crucial element of the work performed to date. At the end of the day, a lot of the health technology challenges that we observe in Ghana will need to be solved by Ghanaian engineers, innovators, and designers. Professor Effah Kaufmann and I have coidentified a need to provide University of Ghana biomedical engineering students with internship opportunities that allow them to gain problem identification and definition experience, and more broadly, engineering design experience. We've found through a research study that there is a mismatch between typical biomedical engineering internships that provide students with experiences more closely aligned with the responsibilities of biomedical technicians and students' perceptions of the discipline formed by watching YouTube videos and reading content on the internet. Many of the Ghanaian biomedical engineering students that I meet are very passionate about innovation and entrepreneurship. As collaborators, Elsie and I have aimed to address this mismatch by providing a subset of the students with an internship opportunity that will allow them to identify unmet needs, define needs, and create solutions. We want to empower the students to take ownership of local needs.

Our numbers are small, but they are intentionally small. It wasn't particularly effective to have ten or more students in the wards of one department at any given point in time because there are nursing students, medical students, and midwifery students also accompanying the medical teams as part of their training. We have to strike a balance of providing non-medical/non-nursing students with these rich clinical experiences while not interfering with patient care or the training of local health care providers.

Therefore, we've decreased our student numbers on the Michigan side and aimed to recruit comparable numbers from the Ghanaian side. We've also promoted peer-to-peer mentoring models. Within

Elsie's classroom, for example, former participants in the clinical immersion and design ethnography experiences share their KBTH design internship perspectives with classmates that haven't had the same experiences. And they challenge their peers to deeply define needs and to use data-driven techniques to define the need.

Our students also stay in contact with one another. We've been intentional in terms of not trying to force-fit a joint capstone design class between our two institutions because we've felt that it would likely fail simply because of the lack of alignment between our institutions' academic calendars. However, our students typically return to Ghana with prototypes during the Ghanaian students' second semester, and they have a chance to reconnect in person as well as critique each other's designs.

Another opportunity that has grown out of the broader UM-Ghana platform is that we've been able to engage graduate-level engineering and non-engineering students in global health design–related activities. One opportunity was through the UM School of Public Health's PARTNER and PARTNER II grants. A second opportunity was through a UM Rackham Graduate School grant that provides mechanical engineering doctoral students with a one-to-two-month internship in Ghana and provides junior faculty in Ghanaian institutions an opportunity to spend one month at UM. In short, we've grown and developed collaborations with Ghanaian partners and trained both UM and Ghanaian students both in Ghana and at UM.

T So you've been able to take what had started as a biomedical platform and really use it and extend it to be an engineering platform.

K Yes, both at the undergraduate and graduate engineering levels. We have also explored relatively new research topics within the field of design science.

T How important do you think it was to have a platform to, to start with?

K As a junior faculty member, the platform was crucial to quickly establishing relationships and initiating new programs. It's hard to imagine being able to accomplish this work without the platform.

K In India I was one of two students that were going out on behalf of our university. And I think a program eventually grew out of our experience.

But I didn't feel like we were plugging into anything. It was a single faculty member that was on the MIT side connecting us with a faculty member at the All-India Institute of Medical Sciences. As students, we were helping to shape a new program through our individual experiences.

T So it was a kind of a one-off make-your-own-adventure story.

K In some ways it was a make-your-own-adventure story. And I think it was a successful make-your-own-adventure story. My understanding is that they formalized the clinical immersion experience after we completed our preceptorship in India. One of the biggest challenges I had as a grad student in India was trying to explain why one needs to have engineers within a clinical environment.

A tremendous benefit of leveraging the Ghana platform was that I did not have to establish foundational university-based partnerships. They existed. I worked with you and others to develop relationships within the existing partnerships. I also absolutely benefitted from senior UM and Ghanaian leaders advocating for me and my new global health design program. We've been at KATH for ten years and the senior leadership understood the value of having engineers in those settings. They've also seen some intangible benefits along the way.

T These are the medical leaders.

K Yes, the leaders within the medical schools.

T Tell me about institutional engagement—you obviously got support from the engineering school and the engineers over there.

K Yes. As you know, we've had particular success with the University of Ghana and KBTH [the University's teaching hospital] partnership. The University of Ghana has a biomedical engineering program, which is a natural fit for global health design work. They're probably one of the oldest biomedical engineering programs in sub-Saharan Africa. We've been working with the University of Ghana and KBTH for the past seven years. And we're in our tenth year of collaborating with KATH [the teaching hospital of Kwame Nkrumah University of Science and Technology in Kumasi]. I'm optimistic that in our tenth year at KATH, we're going to have students from Kwame Nkrumah University of Science and Technology [KNUST]. It's taken longer to find natural partners in engineering at that institution, but I think we're likely to have mechanical engineers participating this summer.

However, it's a good sign that after just a few years of KATH hosting our University of Michigan engineering students, the KATH medical leadership were asking for engagement from KNUST engineering students. In some ways we've been a vehicle to help facilitate local partnerships among Ghanaian institutions.

Although we've gained the support of the senior leaders at KATH and KBTH, there have been challenges along the way in terms of convincing nurses, midwives, and other clinical trainees of the value of having engineering students within the clinical environment. We've learned that it is incredibly important to properly prepare our students prior to the clinical immersion experience. They need to develop clinical literacy and be able to understand basic obstetrics and gynecology terminology. For example, they complete readings and written assignments from an obstetrics and gynecology textbook. They also perform clinical observations at UM on the clinical services, like labor and delivery.

T And that's your story, too, because you had done clinical observations at Harvard Medical School.

K Yes.

T And then you came to Michigan and very quickly had this immersion in, in Ghana.

K Yes.

T And as an engineer, became fluent with language of midwives and obstetrics and words that engineers don't normally use.

K Yes.

T So—and for you, personally, it's been pretty successful. I mean, you've been promoted. You've gotten tenure.

K Yes.

T You're a Thurnau Professor, and now you've expanded past just mechanical engineering and design science. Tell me about this new program.

K We've formalized all these activities under our Global Health Design Initiative [GHDI]. We've benefited from donor support—our students are largely supported by donor funds, and donor funds have recently enabled us to offer paid summer global health design internships.

Last year we supported approximately twenty GHDI students during the time period from March through August.

T And these were not just in Ghana, but other global sites?

K Right. The majority of the students were in Ghana, but we also had students in Ethiopia, Kenya, China, and Nicaragua. Since 2008, we've supported more than 100 international student clinical immersion experiences, with KATH and KBTH as our primary field site partners. We've also engaged more than 350 students in capstone and graduate-level global health design projects.

Most recently, I've cocreated the Center for Socially Engaged Design with two of my Mechanical Engineering colleagues. We are focused on developing educational resources to support engineering students in performing socially engaged design work, with the goal of training them to become lifelong contributors to society through design.

We have an online and asynchronous training academy with learning blocks that students can access on demand, as well as a consultation service. The resources can be used for cocurricular or curricular activities. The learning blocks are coupled with a hands-on skills training session. A lot of the skills that are very important for successful work in the socially engaged design space or the global health design space are non-traditional engineering skills.

For example, how do you conduct effective interviews? How do you perform needs assessments? These are skills that are part and parcel of many non-engineering disciplines. But I personally feel passionate that the engineer needs to be able to perform these activities and be able to communicate as well. Think about a car.

Historically, engineering designers have [been] blind to what marketing has identified as the needs and wants of customers. Engineers have been given information, but it's out of context. They have to use that information to inform design decisions, but they're largely in the dark.

Human- and user-centered design processes and the design-thinking mindset have pushed engineering designers to prioritize stakeholders and end users and to use empathy to understand the needs of various stakeholders. So over the last 20 years, engineers have become more engaged, but they haven't necessarily shaped any of the needs assessments or design ethnography work. But they have some familiarity with the context, and they're starting to value the importance of having these interactions with stakeholders.

I'm pushing for greater involvement—I think it is imperative to have engineers shaping the protocols for the design ethnography work and participating in data collection. An engineer is going to ask different follow-up questions during an interview and make different observations because she or he is going to have to use the data down the road to make design decisions.

I was very interested in getting involved in building socially engaged design educational infrastructure because the lack of resources were and remain a barrier for scaling my global health design work. I liken myself and others in this space to a one-room schoolhouse. There are experts all around our university who can teach these non-traditional engineering topics much better than I can because I haven't been formally trained in these topics. I'm not trained as an anthropologist. I'm not trained as a sociologist. I'm not trained as an obstetrician. We can leverage the skills of others to support the learning process for these students. The hope is that with the infrastructure and physical space in place too, we can start to scale socially engaged design work at the University. The goal is to make some of these resources more broadly available. For example, they could be used to train University of Ghana biomedical engineering students prior to their clinical immersion experience. In the past, we've provided consolidated training materials to the University of Ghana students, but the new platform offers the potential to improve the quality of their training.

T   As you've talked about this, obviously, a lot of this work that you've been doing in Ghana. But for the US, socially engaged design applies to places like Detroit and Flint and Muskegon and, and other under-resourced, low-income, challenged areas in the United States as well, right? A lot of the lessons that you've learned now can apply domestically.

K   Absolutely. There's no reason why the methods in aggregate won't apply to any setting. We've used them for obstetrics and gynecology applications in Ethiopia in addition to Ghana. We've used them in surgical and cancer-related contexts in China. We've also used them in physical medicine and rehabilitation in Kenya. We've also had students use these methods in Nicaragua as part of shorter-term experiences. I'm extremely excited about applying the methods we've been talking about in Flint, Michigan, this summer. We've had to modify the techniques for the time that we have available and adjust for the context of use.

It's interesting for me personally, from a research standpoint, when I reflect on the rehabilitation engineering work that my lab has been doing for balance-related applications in a high-income country context. We had a sort of epiphany a couple of years after applying formal needs identification and problem definition processes in Ghana, because we realized that we weren't using the same methods for design projects aimed at addressing American needs. We were making a lot of design decisions based on assumptions for design projects that had applications within the US context because we felt familiar with the use context. We have grandparents who have balance issues, so we assume we know what their challenges are and what they would need. It's interesting that we had to go to Ghana or Uganda to work on an adult male circumcision device project, where we were completely out of our element, not only from a cultural standpoint, but also from a clinical standpoint, to learn the importance of developing and applying a rigorous front-end design process.

For example, we started using formal needs identification and definition methods when working with older adults in the greater Ann Arbor community, and there's been tremendous benefit to taking time to step back and make sure that our design decisions aren't based on anecdotal information or assumptions, but on data. Unfortunately, we had to learn the lesson while struggling in a different context to see the more local applications of the methods.

T I think this is one of the major lessons that is reinforced in me over and over again when you started doing work in a low-income country. Firstly, people there are so grateful for the work that you do, but then you realize that the multiplier effect is coming back to you in terms of the skills that you acquired and the knowledge that you've learned and the applicability of some of the lessons that are learned in that country that you can apply to your local context. But how do you think the fact that these are academic institution and universities, how does that reverse multiplier work?

K I've benefitted ten- to one-hundred–fold from working with the collaborating partners in Ghana and the student participants, and in unexpected ways. I've been exposed to new fields that have led me down new research pathways and broadened potential funding sources, as well as facilitated my development of expertise in areas that hadn't been part of my core research areas.

The reverse multiplier also serves as an incentive, a daily reminder to look for additional opportunities to make impact within my collaborators' community. It pushes us to think about novel short-term strategies for impact in addition to the longer-term strategies for impact. The most senior clinical collaborators at KBTH and KATH have articulated to me the benefit of having these student trainees perform clinical observations. Certainly, it's a burden on them. It's a burden on their health care system because it's time taken away from the training of other students and from their day-to-day responsibilities. But they've expressed that the time investment is worth it because a subset of the student participants are going to be leaders within the medical device industry in the future. And they will have an eye towards Ghana. They will have an understanding of the use context of medical devices within low-income country settings.

That's one reason why they open their doors and invest their time with the design students. Another reason, and this has taken us five to seven years to recognize, is the culture shift within their department toward a more entrepreneurial mindset from the interactions with the design students. We've increasingly seen senior residents in addition to other clinical trainees proactively identifying unmet needs because they've been working with our undergraduate students and the biomedical engineering students at University of Ghana who are in that setting for the sole purpose of identifying and defining needs. Over the years there has been a shift from having to pull teeth in some cases to get people to talk about the challenges they're encountering to them approaching the students and saying, "Over the last year, we've seen X, Y, and Z. These are real needs. We'd like you to look at these in more depth." Although unintentional, I believe that our students and programs have had a tangible effect on people's day-to-day work. With respect to other forms of short-term impact, I've learned that instructors at other institutions within low-income country settings use the papers that our students have published—for example, the work of Joey Perosky, who was one of our very first engineering students in the GIEU program—as case studies to inform capstone projects and design methodologies within their classrooms.

T   Who is now a medical student.

K   Yes, Joey is now a medical student who has had substantial experience within the global health design space [Andreatta et al., 2012]. Joey's publication about the design of his portable pelvic examination table in the *International Journal for Service Learning in Engineering, Humanitarian Engineering and Social Entrepreneurship* is one example of a student paper that is being used at KNUST within their classroom [Perosky et al., 2012].

We've taken the time to publish the student papers because it is a great experience for the students to contribute to generalizable knowledge. It's nice to see that the descriptions of their design processes are actively being used as teaching instruments.

T   So this is another example of the advantage of being at a university
    because people are actually anxious to publish their papers: publish
    or perish. And scholarship and academics is an important part of the
    process.

K   Yes, I've benefitted from working with academics who are outside of
    my discipline through the UM-Ghana partnerships. As a mechanical
    engineer working in nontraditional mechanical engineering areas,
    I've received a lot of mentorship from faculty outside of engineering.
    I've been encouraged to publish the non-engineering aspects of my
    work, which is something I never would have considered doing if
    I weren't part of this collaborative interdisciplinary group. Through
    our design ethnography work, we not only collect data to inform
    design decisions for various projects, but we collect general cultural
    and contextual data as well. For example, we performed design
    ethnography work in Uganda to better understand traditional adult
    male circumcision processes among four practicing ethnic groups.
    Although we were collecting the data to deeply understand the
    context of the design problem to help inform design decisions for a
    device to protect the glans, we ended up being one of the first groups
    to ever characterize the cutting processes that are used by these four
    ethnic groups. And so we published a qualitative research paper that
    described the four techniques used among these four ethnic groups,
    which was completely outside of my core research area. Again, it goes
    to show that there are a lot of unexpected outcomes of being part of
    this broad platform.

T   I want to ask about interdisciplinary and interprofessional education.
    You're an engineer, but you've worked with medical students. You've
    worked with residents. You've worked with nurses. You've worked
    with midwives. You've worked with psychologists. I mean, you've
    been—you're using anthropologic language here. The GIEU and
    other opportunities here allowed you to bring different groups of
    students together. How do you think that kind of interprofessional
    engagement has worked with the process?

K   I think it's been really important, and we need to move towards more
    formal strategies to train students to work interprofessionally. The

model in the past has been to just bring people together. That is a good start, but we need to be more intentional.

It's been very interesting to watch the evolution of teams with engineering, nursing, and international studies students, for example, as they learn one another's disciplinary languages. We've seen some initial hesitation from the nursing and international studies students to fully engage in the design process, but they eventually learn the design process and contribute in unique ways. I've enjoyed watching them learn about the importance of product requirements and technical specifications, because as engineers, we need to design to meet targets. We need to know whether or not a concept solution will meet the desired product goals.

I've also enjoyed watching the engineering students learn about the complexities associated with the fields of international studies and medicine. They've benefitted from working alongside extremely skilled students from nursing who have the art of the interview down. The nursing school students are adept at engaging with potential stakeholders, and the majority of our engineering students haven't had a chance to develop those same skills through the traditional engineering curriculum. When these students are paired together, the engineer can learn general interviewing skills by example, and the nursing student can learn about interviewing as part of a requirements elicitation process. This type of interprofessional interaction provides a venue for peer-to-peer mentorship across disciplines. And again, we've kind of just let things happen, but I think we can be more intentional moving forward. I think that continuing to develop formal reflection as part of our process will be a step in the right direction. We've built reflection into our programs, but there's more to be done there.

T   And what has been your general approach to trying to equalize the benefits?

K   Yeah. I mean, I think one has to be very intentional to make sure that we reciprocate—that we do for them at least everything that we ask of them to do, we'll do for them. So if we're asking them to take a graduate student, then we'll take a graduate student. If we ask them to take three medical students, then we take three medical students. If we provide funding to send our people over there, we need them to provide funding to bring their people over here. So I mean, we need to be very attentive to economic disparities and inequities and opportunistic inequities because many of our students, by the time they get to be graduate students, have had many more opportunities than theirs have. So we need to be able to enrich this—the experiences of the students from low-income countries who often have not had the opportunities that our students have. This is the greatest challenge for me at this point. It's what keeps me up at night. Fairness. We try to approach fairness with a multifaceted perspective because "one-for-one" exchanges don't always work.

T And I think the Charter principles are important that you mentioned. I've been thinking more and more about kind of the, the ethics of global health. And I think you're now talking about the ethics of global biomedical engineering, right?

K Yes, there are numerous ethical considerations with respect to the undergraduate and graduate educational opportunities that we've been discussing, and we need to continue to carefully address these issues as our partnerships grow.

Lessons Learned

Innovation is reproducible.

Academic opportunities are often reproducible across disciplines.

Faculty development in education and research builds academic capacity.

When someone knocks on your door, answer it quickly.

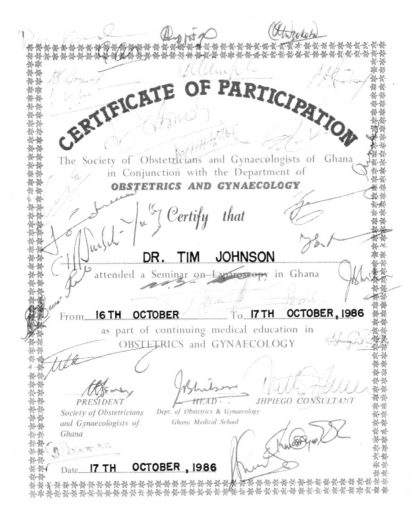

CERTIFICATE OF PARTICIPATION

The Society of Obstetricians and Gynaecologists of Ghana
in Conjunction with the Department of
OBSTETRICS AND GYNAECOLOGY

Certify that

DR. TIM JOHNSON

attended a Seminar on Laparoscopy in Ghana

From **16 TH OCTOBER**   To **17 TH OCTOBER, 1986**

as part of continuing medical education in
OBSTETRICS and GYNAECOLOGY

PRESIDENT   _HEAD_   _JHPIEGO CONSULTANT_
Society of Obstetricians   _Dept. of Obstetrics & Gynaecology_
and Gynaecologists of   _Ghana Medical School_
Ghana

Date **17 TH OCTOBER , 1986**

Figure 1 Certificate of Attendance of the Society of Obstetricians and
Gynecologists of Ghana conference in 1986 signed by attendees. This event was
the stimulus for the development of the Ghana Postgraduate Training Programme
in Obstetrics and Gynaecology.

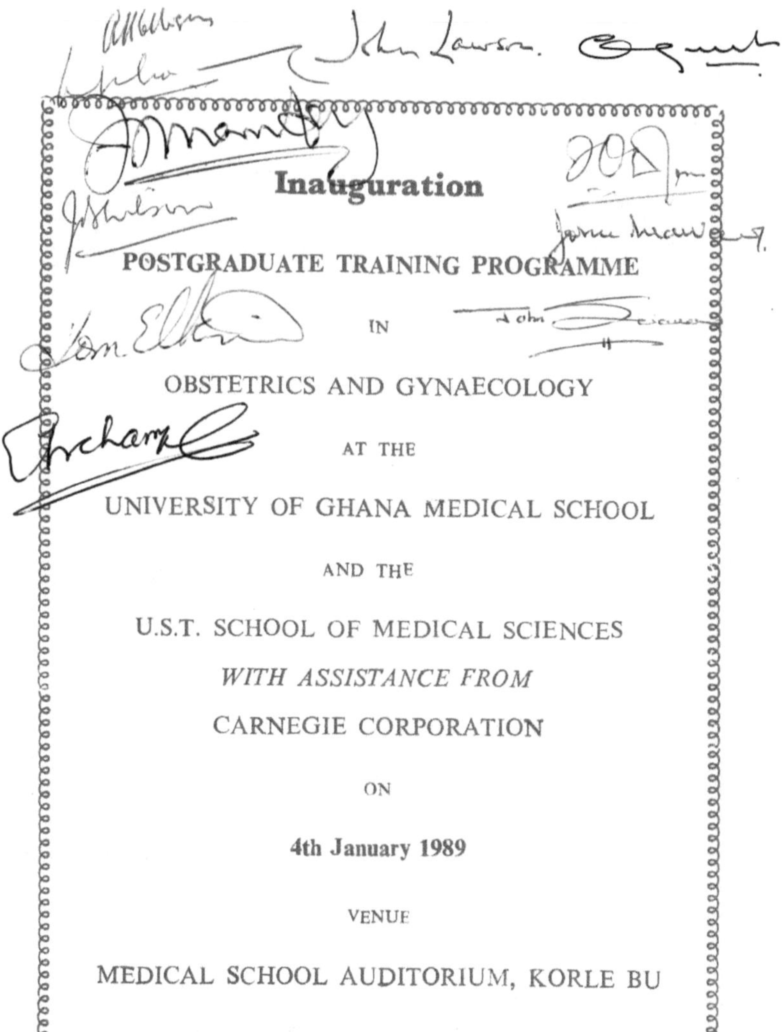

Inauguration

POSTGRADUATE TRAINING PROGRAMME

IN

OBSTETRICS AND GYNAECOLOGY

AT THE

UNIVERSITY OF GHANA MEDICAL SCHOOL

AND THE

U.S.T. SCHOOL OF MEDICAL SCIENCES

WITH ASSISTANCE FROM

CARNEGIE CORPORATION

ON

4th January 1989

VENUE

MEDICAL SCHOOL AUDITORIUM, KORLE BU

Figure 2 Inauguration program for the launch of the Ghana Postgraduate Training Programme in Obstetrics and Gynecology signed by the External Advisory Board members.

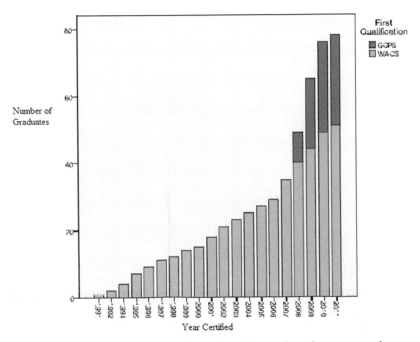

Figure 3 Graph showing the annual growth in the number of program graduate from 1991 to present.

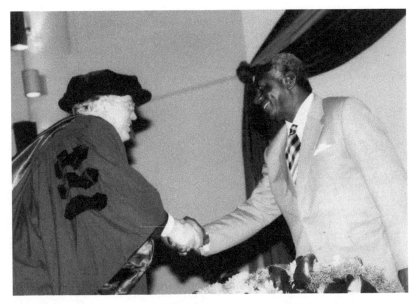

Figure 4 Doctor Johnson congratulated by Ghana President John Kufuor on becoming honorary Fellow of the Ghana College of Physicians and Surgeons.

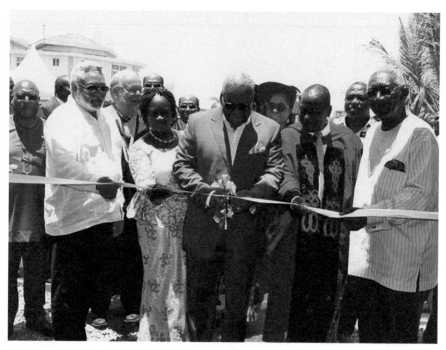

Figure 5 Ribbon cutting for the opening of the Family Health University College Medical School. Front row: former Ghana President Jerry Rawlings (white shirt) Minister of Education, President John Mahama, Founding Dean & Professor Yao Kwawukume, former President John Kufour; second row in academic robes Doctor Timothy Johnson and Founding COO/Doctor Susu Kwawukume.

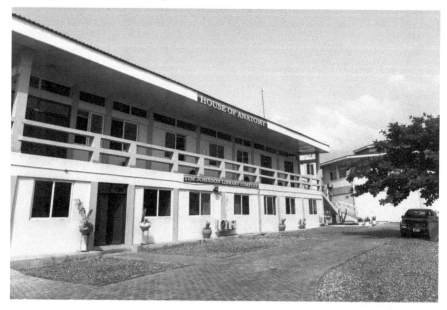

Figure 6 Tim Johnson Library Complex in the Anatomy Building on the Family Health University College campus.

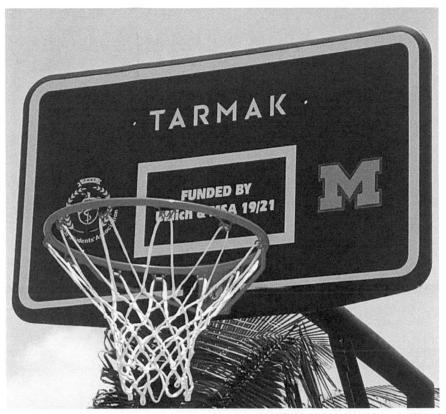

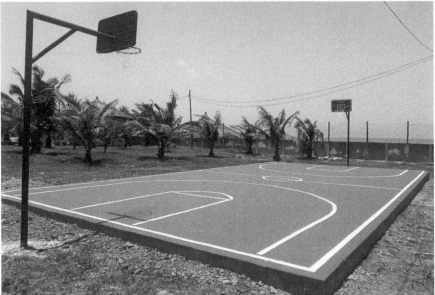

Figure 7 Basketball court on the Family Health University College campus with the Atlantic Ocean in the background and built with support of the Ghana Medical Student Association and the University of Michigan GLOBAL REACH.

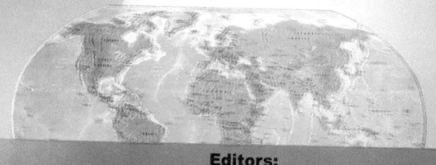

Comprehensive
Obstetrics
In The Tropics

Editors:
E. Y. Kwawukume
B. A. Ekele
K. A. Danso
E. Ejiro Emuveyan

Figure 8 Cover of *Comprehensive Obstetrics in the Tropics*, the first obstetric text
published by an all-African author team for use in Sub-Saharan Africa.

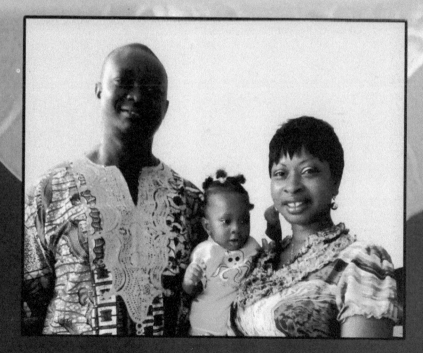

COMPREHENSIVE REPRODUCTIVE HEALTH AND FAMILY PLANNING IN THE TROPICS

Editors: K.A Danso, E.Y Kwawukume, H. Tagbor, R.K.O Asante
Inauagural Fellows: D.Z. Kobilla, E.S.K. Morhe, E.T. Maya, K. Mumuni

Figure 9 Cover of <u>Comprehensive Reproductive Health and Family Planning in the Tropics</u>, published by faculty and fellows in the Reproductive Health and Family Planning fellowship for use in Ghana and across Sub-Saharan Africa.

FIRST BATCH OF EMERGENCY MEDICINE RESIDENTS ADMITTED

The first batch of residents for the Membership programme in Emergency Medicine has been admitted. The College's Emergency Medicine programme is run at the Komfo Anokye Teaching Hospital with support from the University of Michigan and the University of Utah.

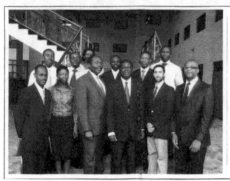

With the 8 residents who were interviewed for admission are Professor Paul Nyame, Rector of the Ghana College of Physicians and Surgeons. Dr. Conrad Buckle (1st from right), Dr. Daniel Wachter (2nd from right) and Dr. George Oduro (3rd from left) are all Emergency Medicine Specialists who will be part of the Faculty to help with the training.

Figure 10 "First batch" of Emergency Medicine residents highlighted by the Ghana College of Physicians and Surgeons.

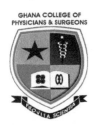

GHANA COLLEGE OF PHYSICIANS AND SURGEONS

&

UNIVERSITY OF MICHIGAN

Present

A Pre-Conference Workshop of the 6th Annual General and Scientific Meeting on

FAMILY MEDICINE SEMINAR

Date: Tuesday, 8th December, 2009

Time: 08.00 am to 4.00 pm

Venue: Ghana College of Physicians and Surgeons,

54, Independence Avenue, Ridge, Accra

Figure 11 Family Medicine seminar sponsored by the Ghana College of Physicians and Surgeons.

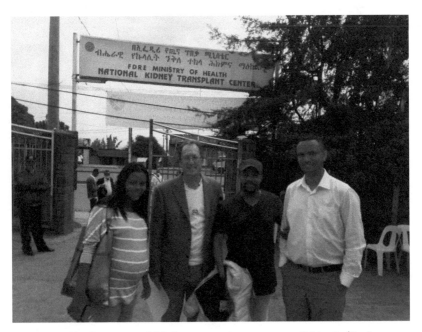

Figure 12 The first successful kidney transplant patient in Ethiopia (Berhanu, third from left), after his recovery, with his pregnant wife, Doctor Jeffrey Punch, and Ethiopian surgeon Doctor Engida Abebe who assisted in the surgery.

Locating Culture with/in a Ghanaian Community

Raymond Silverman
University of Michigan

Techiman is the capital of Bono, Ghana's earliest state. It is also the site of Ghana's largest agricultural market. Today, Techiman is a cosmopolitan community comprised of peoples from all over West Africa. Here, "culture" is perceived as Bono heritage and Bono chiefs serve as its custodians.

Roughly ten years ago the Traditional Council of Chiefs of Techiman launched an initiative to create a cultural center to celebrate Bono heritage. It has been a fraught but productive process. The project has evolved to include the multiple heritages of Techiman's diverse population and to engage members of the community in the planning process. Recent collaborative efforts involving community leaders working with scholars and students from several Ghanaian and Michigan universities have established "heritage dialogues" that encourage the citizens of the town to think about the cultures of Techiman—where are these diverse traditions located and how might they be presented and shared in a new institution that offers a physical place and a social space for the performance and preservation of culture?

The project has profound implications for establishing and sustaining a social and political identity for Techiman, as well as for its constituent communities. The process of creating the cultural center is fostering democratic practice and strengthening civil society in Techiman. This paper explores the dynamics of this collaborative "culturework," focusing primarily on how engaging a community in thinking about its heritage(s) can serve as a catalyst for social and political change.

lecture
Tuesday, January 12, 7:00 pm
Stern Auditorium, Lower Level, UM Museum of Art

workshop
Wednesday, January 13, 4:00-5:30 pm
Multi-Purpose Room, First Floor, UM Museum of Art

Free and open to the public

This lecture and workshop are part of the Museum Studies Program year-long colloquium,
Translating Knowledge: Global Perspectives on Museum and Community.

Cosponsored by the African Studies Center, Arts of Citizenship, Bentley Historical Library, Center for Afroamerican and African Studies, Center for South Asian Studies, Center for Southeast Asian Studies, Department of Anthropology, Doctoral Program in Anthropology and History, Eisenberg Institute for Historical Studies, Exhibit Museum of Natural History, Institute for the Humanities, International Institute, LS&A Theme Semester, Office of the President, Office of the Provost, Native American Studies, Pacific Islands Workshop, U-M Museum of Anthropology, and U-M Museum of Art.

MUSEUM STUDIES PROGRAM
UNIVERSITY OF MICHIGAN ■ ANN ARBOR

www.umich.edu/~ummsp ■ 734.936.6678 ■ ummsp@umich.edu

Figure 13 Announcement of a Museum Studies program on building a cultural center in Techiman, Ghana organized in Ann Arbor by Professor Ray Silverman.

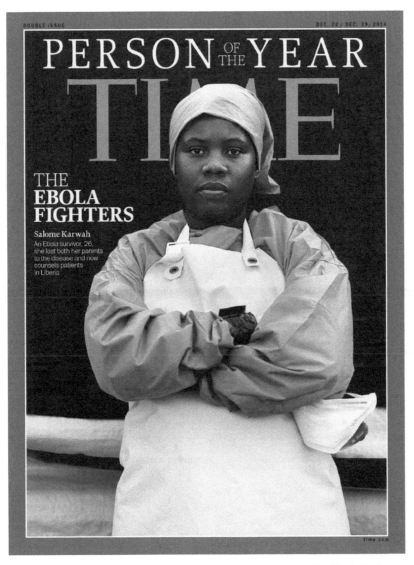

Figure 14 Person of the Year cover of Time magazine, 2014, The Ebola Fighters, represented by Salome Karwah, a nurse who survived Ebola but later died of preventable, treatable blood pressure complications of pregnancy.

CHAPTER 10

Reproducibility and Replication: Ethiopia

Once the GPTP was established, and especially after the presentation by Professor Klufio at the National Association of Professors of Gynecology and Obstetrics (APGO) meeting (Klufio et al., 2003), the comments we heard recurrently were: "This is a unique situation," "It could only work in Ghana," "It only worked because of the Carnegie funding," and "It could never work in our institution." As this book attempts to show, this work in academic global health is reproducible. One of my favorite aphorisms about innovation, change, and disruptive ideas, attributed to Henry James, is: "First they say it is not true. Then they say it is not important. Then they say it is not new."

An example from my Michigan experience might be clarifying, with its perspective on innovation and change from a different lens. Early after my arrival at University of Michigan, it was no surprise that the medical malpractice issue was an important concern and frequent topic of conversation in the Department of Obstetrics and Gynecology. The department had a history of major lawsuits and large settlements, and cases were pending that were concerning. In meetings with legal office colleagues, several major areas of exposure were identified and targeted for early identification at the time of the event—with immediate reporting, case investigation, root cause analysis, and a culture of "not to blame the individual." Major areas of concern were perinatal events (low Apgar scores, birth asphyxia, etc.), twins, preterm delivery, shoulder dystocia, failure to diagnose cancer (gynecologic and breast), and management of ectopic pregnancy including diagnosis and surgery timing. These turned out to be exactly the major issues we subsequently faced, and the focus served us well over twenty years and probably will inform low-income countries for the future as physician responsibility and patient safety become more important. All major clinical conditions are universal; the major diseases afflicting people, and women specifically, are essentially similar everywhere in the world. As part of this early recognition medicolegal paradigm, we included early meetings to debrief the team and collect information close to the adverse event. Patients were made aware of these events, and a culture of full disclosure to patients became more and more institutionalized. Patients who were harmed due to medical error were compensated immediately. There was no required proscription of malpractice suits, but patients who have been fully informed about their medical care and trust that they have been treated with the full honesty, we demonstrated, are less likely to sue. Soon, "disclosure" became part of the policy and practice at University of Michigan Health System (UMHS) and was popularized by our senior lawyer partner in the process, Richard Boothman (Kachalia et al., 2010). It was cited as a best practice by Hilary Clinton and Barack Obama in an editorial on health care reform in the *New England Journal of Medicine* (Clinton & Obama, 2006). Medical malpractice claims dropped across UMHS and have remained low with the disclosure policy that is in place and continually enhanced. Many people said this innovative practice and policy was not reproducible; that it could only be done at the University of Michigan, or in Ann Arbor, or in Michigan, or at a public university's academic medical center. People were unwilling to accept this radical new way of dealing with medical errors, hospital events, or sometimes even just patient perceptions of events that were not necessarily abnormal or linked to poor outcome.

Time and experience across the United States have shown that others who tried disclosure found similar results. Universally telling patients the truth early and candidly actually made them better connected with medical providers and found them less likely to sue. This was an important morality tale for me, and the ethical implications have been felt by visiting Ghanian medical students, residents, and faculty. They have come to understand and embrace the commonly repeated phrase "The Michigan Difference."

Just as in the "disclosure" example, many American and international academic colleagues thought and said that the GPTP example was not reproducible; that Ghana was "special"; that the timing was uniquely important for the success; that the Carnegie funding or the RCOG or ACOG involvement was critical and necessary for success. Was the GPTP model reproducible? Could it be replicated by other institutions and in and between other countries?

The answer is yes, as demonstrated by the great success of the application of the Ghana program model to health care capacity building in Ethiopia. In 1998, I spoke with a terrific young resident applicant, Senait Fisseha, who was receiving her MD and JD from Southern Illinois University, and convinced her that since she was interested in global work, Michigan was the place for her to come for residency. She did brilliantly as a resident, did a three-year subspecialty fellowship in reproductive endocrinology and infertility, and then joined the faculty, rising to chief of the Division of Reproductive Endocrinology and Infertility.

As a resident, Doctor Fisseha experienced a month's rotation in Ghana. She grew up in Ethiopia, and one of the reasons she came to UM for residency was because of the potential to participate global women's health experiences. Opportunity again favored a prepared mind.

In Ethiopia, as the minister of health starting in 2005, Doctor Tedros Adhanom Ghebreyesus developed a strategy for creating more medical schools to create more doctors to "flood" the country with these trained doctors and provide universal health coverage and services to all people, even in the most remote areas. He received worldwide recognition as young Ethiopian doctors did indeed spread across the country and contributed meaningfully to Ethiopia's notable and almost unique success in approaching all and achieving many of the UN Millennium Development Goals (MDGs) of 2015 (See table).

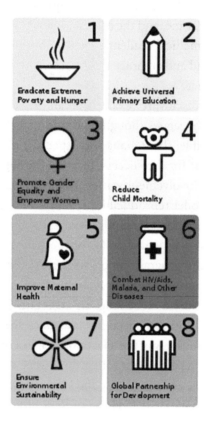

Many from this burgeoning medical workforce, after two to three years of national service in outlying health centers, wanted to then become specialized in such fields as surgery, cardiology, and OBGYN. Doctor Tedros (Ethiopian common usage is to use a first name as a form of address) was a PhD epidemiologist and a scientist, so he looked to the published literature to identify successful international post-graduate specialty training programs—programs that were sustainable and local—and through our publications (Klufio et al., 2003; Anderson et al., 2007; Clinton et al., 2010) he "found" the Ghana-UM program. He spoke with Doctor Fisseha, who was known to him through Ethiopian diaspora contacts, and made a special side trip to Ann Arbor when he was in the United States to receive an award from the Clinton Foundation for his work on physician capacity building in Ethiopia through the "flooding policy." When he met with Doctor Fisseha, Dean Joe Kolars, and me, he said, "I want this program in Ethiopia." He said to me, "I want YOU to bring this program to Ethiopia." I repeated with emphasis that Ghana was the country I had committed to, but I would be happy to support, mentor, and work with Doctor Fisseha to develop OBGYN training in Ethiopia. Her rock-star achievements were highlighted in the *Lancet* (Lane, 2019). Her intelligence, passion, excellent preparatory on-the-ground experience in Ghana, and the resources that Doctor Tedros made available allowed her to quickly and efficiently develop the OBGYN and other residency training programs in Ethiopia.

With support from the CDC and the Ethiopian MOH (remember THAT lesson), Doctor Fisseha began her intensive work at a single institution, St. Paul's Hospital Millennium Medical College. SPHMMC was a new medical school and new academic medical center envisioned by Doctor Tedros. It would be a center of excellence for women's health, and a brand-new teaching hospital for women's and children's health was planned for its campus. SPHMMC was also unique in that it was set up as the first medical school in Ethiopia with a modular curriculum established to train doctors to serve the country. National service, universal health care, and primary health care for all parts of the country, especially the rural areas, were institutionalized under Doctor Tedros's plans. At the onset, there was no residency training program affiliated with SPHMMC. Doctor Fisseha was in the country giving lectures on cervical cancer screening and prevention (much like my initial talk in Ghana that led to GPTP) and, in another "but for" situation, met with Doctor Lia Tadesse, a trained OBGYN who was vice-provost of SPHMMC, and the idea of residency training programs coalesced. It had previously been discussed locally with Doctor Tedros—once again, opportunity collided with intention and a prepared mind. Doctor Fisseha had experienced the Ghana model in action during her residency rotation there. She saw SPHMMC as an immediate opportunity to address the very high burden of maternal mortality in Ethiopia and implement the Safe Motherhood Initiative. At the time, Addis Ababa University and teaching hospitals at the universities in Jimma and Gondar were the only residency training programs in Ethiopia. Doctor Fisseha saw the by-now established Ghana model as an evidence-based implementation program and a possible South-South partnership for Ethiopia. South-South partnerships, where universities in the low- and middle-income countries of the Global South exchange intellectual and human resource capacity, have long been an idea and a proposed ideal in global health. Doctor Fisseha arranged a visit to Ethiopia by Doctor Richard Adanu from Ghana, Rani Kotha, an experienced program manager, and me, representing Michigan's GLOBAL REACH team. After that first visit in February 2011, Doctor Lia Tadesse came to Ann Arbor for a planning visit. At the time, Doctor Lia and Doctor Abdulfetah were the only OBGYN faculty at SPHMMC. An initial competency-based residency curriculum was developed by SPHMMC faculty and medical education staff, with input from Doctor Senait, RCOG, the established and world-famous Black Lion (Tikur Anbessa) Specialized Hospital affiliated with Addis Ababa University, and UM.

A residency with two faculty was started shortly thereafter, with the hope of luring two to five more faculty from other institutions (another "reverse brain drain" opportunity) and recruiting graduating students from SPHMMC. The rapid success and expansion of the program is shown by this timeline:

Program launched in June 2012
2012: 7 residents (all graduated in 2016, by then 16 faculty)
2013: 14 residents (12 graduated in 2017)
2014: 15 residents (12 graduated in 2018)
2015: 31 residents (2 from South Sudan)
2016: 28 residents started
2017: 25 residents expected

Fellowships soon followed, with maternal-fetal medicine starting in 2014 (Doctor Abdulfetah had also trained as a subspecialist in MFM in Germany), followed by fellowships in family planning , gynecologic oncology, and reproductive endocrinology and infertility. These programs all accepted two incoming fellows per year and were three-year programs. The first MFM fellows graduated in 2017 and took positions at SPHMMC and, subsequently, other teaching hospitals throughout the country. In addition to OBGYN, Doctor Fisseha was also instrumental in starting residency programs at SPHMMC in general surgery in 2014, then in internal medicine; radiology; anesthesia; pediatrics, with substantial help from colleagues at Tulane; and ophthalmology, with significant help from colleagues at the Jerome Jacobson International Program at the Kellogg Eye Center at the University of Michigan (Heisel et al., 2020, 2021).

This expansion of training offerings was another of Doctor Tedros's "visions." Along with the leadership of SPHMMC, he wanted very intentionally to develop programs that could compete with those offered at Black Lion Hospital, which had long been the premier teaching and training hospital in Ethiopia. Doctor Tedros felt that everyone would benefit from friendly competition to limit any tendency for complacency among the rising number of medical schools and teaching hospitals in Ethiopia. He saw healthy competition as good, and Doctor Lia and Doctor Fisseha were nothing if not competitive. One unique program established at SPHMMC was the first renal transplant program in Ethiopia (Punch, 2023). Initially, there was a critically important onsite evaluation and preparation by UM transplant nephrologist Doctor Alan Leichtman. Laboratory and perioperative capacity were enhanced to world-class standards. This included the construction of a brand-new, totally modern, freestanding transplant center. A medical team to manage the long-term immunosuppression required for the transplant recipients was also developed. Doctor Jeff Punch, a senior UM transplant surgeon, worked with the Ethiopia team to train extensively and then perform the first renal transplant in Ethiopia in 2015. At the time they were performing four cases in batches, using living related-donor kidneys, over a small number of days to optimize perioperative and postoperative care, which was all accomplished at the transplant center. By 2017 there had been about forty transplants, and the Ethiopia team now performs these transplants independent of outside presence and assistance. I find this an informative and inspiring model for the introduction of a life-saving, formerly "high-tech, high-income country" technology to almost anywhere in the world.

One of my favorite images of the capacity of global health for good is a very personal one. The very first transplant, to everyone's satisfaction (and relief), turned out to be entirely successful for a young man who was near death from renal failure and received a living family-donor transplant. After a successful recovery, he returned to a regular life, married, and brought his pregnant wife with him for a photo with Doctor Punch and Doctor Engida Abebe, his Ethiopian colleague and transplant surgeon, in front of the Kidney Transplant Center of Ethiopia.

Doctor Punch continues to mentor the Ethiopian transplant surgeons he helped train, is currently working to develop transplant capacity in Kenya and Rwanda, and continues to visit Ethiopia on occasion, even though he had a near-fatal heart attack while operating with his colleagues on one of the early transplants. He stepped back from the operating table and fell to the floor unconscious. Luckily, he was surrounded by competent physicians and was resuscitated and transported to the newly constructed specialized cardiology center in Addis Ababa, where he recovered. When he returned to Ann Arbor, cardiac catheterization showed he needed coronary artery stenting. I have no doubt that minimally invasive coronary artery therapy was soon on the wish list of the Ethiopian Ministry of Health, where Doctor Lia Tadesse is now minister of health.

With this Ethiopia program, SPHMMC and MOH addressed a pressing need: training postgraduates in key selected areas to address basic issues such as an excessive rate of maternal mortality and morbidity, to meet other Safe Motherhood Initiative goals. It also met other increasingly desirable health care needs, such as pediatrics, cardiology, ophthalmology, and aligned institutional needs with country priorities. To note, there was substantial female leadership in this program from Doctor Fisseha to Doctor Tadesse's vision for a planned mother and children's health specialty hospital, which just recently opened as a spectacular modern hospital. From the onset Doctor Mesfin, the SPHMMC provost, committed to academic growth, demonstrating commitment to faculty development, especially woman faculty. Doctor Adanu returns regularly to Ethiopia for introductory and advanced research training sessions.

Doctor Fisseha has always inspired people, not just people at UM but people in Ethiopia: students, residents, faculty, and representatives from MOH both during and after Doctor Tedros's tenure as minister. Faculty development at SPHMMC was very important and intentional. Bilateral exchanges with Michigan showed Ethiopians differences in how medicine was practiced in the United States. Like the Ghanaians, Ethiopians were struck by the patient-centered approach to care and the involvement of patients in shared decision making. Operational issues such as patient flow, team operations, patient and team communication, 360-degree evaluations (with unit clerks, nurses, students, residents, and faculty all evaluating each other) were carefully observed, and some parts were no doubt taken back for integration into the Ethiopian medical education and health care culture. In 2013 SPHMMC began requiring in-house faculty presence, an American practice dating from the 1980s, after Ethiopian visitors had seen the advantages of this policy on the quality and safety of patient care and on the education and training of residents and students. Ethiopian visitors saw UM residents involved with research projects through local presentations and at national meetings. Resident research was expected from the start of the SPHMMC residency and, as we have stated, Professor Richard Adanu from Ghana provided intensive research training for faculty in Years 1 and 2, and now provides regular workshops for faculty and residents.

Doctor Balkachew, the OBGYN residency program director at SPHMMC, attended the US Council on Resident Education in Obstetrics and Gynecology (CREOG) meetings and introduced a virtual model of the popular CREOG "program director's school," a virtual must-do for American program directors, to Ethiopia in 2016. Attended by residency program directors and aspiring program directors from across the country, this was a great example of national institution building using an international (CREOG) model.

One impact on the SPHMMC medical school was the development of a strong focus on family planning and contraception, with skills learned in implementation of long-acting reversible contraception (LARC) and safe abortion. The first SPHMMC graduates in community and rural National Service practice demonstrably participated in reproductive health services, established family planning services, and assumed leadership roles in quality care initiatives or as medical directors with their recently learned skills. Simulation training and leadership training were introduced in the medical school—like simulation and leadership additions to all contemporary US curricula—although this time they were adopted early in the development of the residency training that spread across Ethiopia.

The program also served to increase the international visibility of Doctor Fisseha (Lane, 2019). As the program developed, she received a large grant to expand this comprehensive competency-based reproductive health and family planning training to all the medical schools in Ethiopia. Within one year, the foundation she was working with was so happy with the progress of her programs and her successful vision that she was recruited to be the director of global programs at the foundation headquarters. While she kept an adjunct appointment at the University of Michigan, she moved on to become one of the major financial agents and visionaries in creating opportunities for global women's health in the world. This was certainly a very satisfying career path for a faculty member at Michigan with global women's health interests. She continues this work, being very involved with a variety of foundations including the Bill & Melinda Gates Foundation, the Clinton Foundation, and others, and is working closely with WHO, International Planned Parenthood Foundation, and other major organizations to focus on the priorities of the private foundation. She is also a special counsel to Doctor Tedros, who has become director-general of the WHO.

The rapid proliferation of residencies In Ethiopia demonstrates the kinds of things that can happen with a plan, a vision, some additional economic support, and the engagement of local clinicians who are committed to rapid change and capacity building. All this reflects the confident belief that what could happen in Ghana could happen in Ethiopia, even though it was a much larger and very different country. Unlike the approach that occurred in Ghana at two excellent medical schools with established teaching hospitals, Ethiopia saw a modified approach applied to a single nascent medical school with a transitioning teaching hospital that quickly became a national center of excellence for postgraduate obstetrics and gynecology training and, ultimately, the clinical headquarters for the Center for International Reproductive Health Training (supported by the foundation where Doctor Fisseha was based) that was focused on developing capacity in RHFP for medical students and trainees across Ethiopia, with the goal of ultimately transferring its model across the world.

In many ways, the success in Ethiopia was based on the Ghana program, except that what took eight years in Ghana only took four years in Ethiopia, simply because there was experience and a track record of what worked in the African context. There was a blueprint based on the publications that existed, and the kinds of support that was needed were known. In addition, there was support from the Ministry of Health, the developing new medical school, and all the things that Doctor Fisseha learned both at Michigan from the Ghana programs we had specifically developed and from her own specific Ethiopian knowledge base. Once again, the program in Ethiopia was a combination of the American ideas, since the faculty knew about the Ghana legacy and had attended APGO/CREOG and other American professional society meetings, but it also was culturally reflective to the types of change happening in Ethiopia, which has previously been a more Eurocentric model. One difference was the fellowships that were created, which look very much like the US model, with training in subspecialties such as family planning and reproductive health, gynecologic oncology, maternal-fetal medicine, urogynecology in obstetrics and gynecology, and subsequently, training in other departments as well.

Doctor Fisseha has summarized her experience with the Michigan model of global health this way:

> I came to the University of Michigan for the first time in 1998. I came to interview for residency and during my interview met Doctor Tim Johnson. At that time, I knew I wanted to be involved in global health and, particularly at, be at some point in my career involved in Ethiopia.

When I came to interview and shared that vision with Tim, he was able to help me crystalize my thoughts and in very simple terms explained to me how he saw global health. He clearly articulated to me how he sees collaboration as a strength and that he always advises people to focus on one country; when you have a relationship, it has to be a long-term relationship and you keep on coming back. You are there when the going gets tough. You were there at all times. You build relationships that are bilateral and mutually beneficial. He relayed the principles. In these simple terms he explained to me how he saw global health.

In my years at Michigan, that started when I was a resident, so essentially after that conversation I stopped looking anywhere else for my residency and decided to come to Michigan. I came here, finished a very busy intern year, and right at the end of my intern year, I think the first month of my second-year residency, started in Ghana. I spend one month in Ghana. I went with another resident friend of mine, and we spent one month. The moment we got there we were able to feel Doctor Johnson's presence. Because he had built such positive relationships we were seen in his light. We were treated very well. We were treated like a colleague. We were expected to be involved. We were treated like we were long-term collaborators although it was our first time there. When I was there, I met residents and when I came back [to] Ann Arbor those residents came to Michigan. So as Tim had said, it was not a one-way street, it was bidirectional and bilateral. It was mutually beneficial. We were going there to gain experience and residents from Ghana were coming to Michigan.

My third year at Michigan, one of the senior residents from Ghana came to spend his time at Michigan, and this was Richard Adanu, who is now the dean of the School of Public Health of the University of Ghana. What Tim has been able to build and what we really dub as the "Michigan Difference" is this long-term collaboration that is constant, that is mutually beneficial, that builds on the work that has been done but it continues to evolve to not only reflect the past but also to meet the needs of the current time and also anticipate the needs of the future. The Michigan-Ghana collaboration evolved from building capacity of obstetricians/gynecologists to collaboration on research and having watched that for so many, many years. When it was time for me to start building my Ethiopia relationship, it was very easy to transport that culture of the Michigan-Ghana collaboration to the Michigan-Ethiopia model. The Michigan-Ethiopia collaboration is really built on the platform that Tim built for Ghana, and we essentially took that "charter for collaboration" that was built on mutual benefit and transparency and openness and shared responsibility and brought that culture, but not only that culture of the Michigan collaboration, but we also brought our partners from Ghana to build a collaboration in Ethiopia. It really has been a very remarkable journey and one that I will look back upon and will always be grateful for the day that I walked in Tim Johnson's office, not only for the things that I have been able to benefit from directly or being able to do in Ethiopia but the ability to work with a person who has this huge vision for the world. A transformative vision and a vision that is inclusive of everyone. This has been an asset for me. That is my short take on the Michigan way of collaboration.

I asked Doctor Lia Tadesse to permit me to do a narrative interview about her perspective of the development and success of the SPHMMC. At the time of the initiation of the SPHMMC program, she was an OBGYN who had been appointed vice-provost of SPHMMC. The interview was done at the time she was in Ann Arbor directing the nascent Center for International Reproductive Health Training. Upon her return to Ethiopia, she entered the Ministry of Health and shortly after was named Minister of Health:

T (Tim Johnson) This is Tim Johnson and I'm here with Doctor Lia Tadesse to talk about the beginnings of the Ethiopia program. How do you remember first hearing about the possibility of a new training program? You were provost of Millennium St. Paul Medical School [sic]. What existed at the time? Was there an OB and GYN residency training program?

L (Lia Tadesse) No, I was vice-provost, focused on the medical services initially, and St. Paul was a new medical school, which was established in 2007. This work started in 2011. St. Paul's, the school itself, was primarily an initiative of the minister of health, specifically Doctor

Tedros's initiative to produce a new kind of physician workforce really coming from all parts of the country and also willing to serve their country. It had a different recruitment process than the usual medical school. We had an also, kind of a different curriculum, which was a modular integrated curriculum. St. Paul's, as a new medical school, even though the hospital was full, it was growing at the time, just building up to be a strong medical school. And we didn't have any residency program at the time.

We had started to talk with potential partners. One of the partners we had was an Ethiopian North American Health Professionals Association. They had arranged a conference regarding women's cancer at the African Union, where Doctor Senait Fisseha had come to present about cervical cancer. So she had been working closely with eight to ten North American institutions. She had played a big part working with that association for years before that. I attended that conference. And the people from the North American Association introduced me and Senait at the time. It was a wonderful opportunity to meet with her. I'd heard about her from them before. So we started talking about the program at St. Paul and the interests. And she also had been for the years before that visiting Ethiopia. Just a few weeks or months after we met, she invited Doctor Tedros to come to the University of Michigan to visit with the department. So that's when he visited there and met all the faculty there and arranged for some of their faculty to visit Ethiopia and St. Paul. One thing is he had these big plans for St. Paul to grow as an academic institution, for he knew this would require strong, strong work, especially the physicians. There was a big maternal mortality in Ethiopia, which was still showing not much progress, despite the progress in child mortality.

T   So it seems safe motherhood was an important issue—

L   It was a very important issue. And despite that, the number of residency programs in OBGYN in the whole country were low. Black Lion Teaching Hospital of Addis Ababa University was the longstanding one. But at the time, there were two more, at Gondar and Jimma. Yes. So there was a very strong interest to expand the OBGYN workforce. So when Tedros came to Michigan, he really wanted to expand residencies, and he saw the work that had [been] done with Ghana. He was really interested in that, in that collaboration which shows how the capacity building has impacted the Ghana program. So he really wanted University of Michigan to support specifically St. Paul's, to do the same thing and start OBGYN residency and continue the other related initiatives—

T I guess Tedros, first of all, was a prepared mind.

L Yes.

T But he's also an academic. And so when he saw the Ghana program had been successful, he saw an opportunity to kind of replicate that in Ethiopia, right?

L In Ethiopia. Yeah. Absolutely. And having some nice work for Michigan colleagues to do something for Ethiopia here in Ann Arbor, too—

T It, it worked out.

L It worked out. So we didn't feel an immediate effect of his visit. But soon we were very fortunate to have you and, of course, Doctor Senait, Doctor Richard Adanu, from Ghana, and this was, I think, a first time we were all able to meet together.

T We all came together at the visit, that's when we met and kind of brainstormed on the possibility of starting this residency program. And was that in 2011?

L It was 2011, yeah. It was the same time.

T So it all happened—I mean, this all happened very quickly.

L Very quickly. So that was, I think, February 2011 and then, May 2011, I actually came for the first visit to the University of Michigan to make a first connection. So and then immediately after that—well, at that time, the only OBGYN faculty that St. Paul had was my junior colleague. I was not working much on the clinical side because I was more in the administrative work. There was only one practicing OBGYN there. Of course, we had Black Lion faculty, faculty from the other university coming on-site. So other than that, it was one person on-site, teaching students.

T So you had visiting faculty from Black Lion?

L From Black Lion, yes.

T How much the world has changed. [By the time of this interview, faculty had left Black Lion for SPHMMC and Black Lion was short-staffed.]

L I know. It has—it has gone so far now. So at the time, we started working with some other doctors, saying "Okay. Now, let's start working." It seemed like a crazy idea to even think of establishing an OBG residency program with only two faculty, with only one or two people. But we were really hopeful to be able to get others, especially considering that this collaboration with Michigan would be there with the potential for faculty development in terms of the development of the St. Paul Millennial Medical School—

T To lure—you were really going to lure new faculty.

L Yeah. So, so we started searching for potential interested faculty. And that's how we got to get the first three faculty to come.

T So, Doctor Balkachew.

L And Doctor Delayehu were the ones we recruited. And then, there were—Delayehu was working at an NGO [non-governmental organization, usually supported with external funds and externally determined projects and leadership], and Balkachew was working at a private hospital. But they were both interested in academia. And they had been in academia before that and had gone to private hospitals and an NGO, primarily for private financial funding.

T You knew people like this were out there?

L Yeah. So they were really interested to come back to academia, and especially when we discussed with them the partnership of Michigan, they were excited about a place which was newly starting OBGYN residency and talking about building a new maternity and women's hospital.

T Okay. So soon you had three: Obkofana, Balkachew, and Delayehu.

LR Yes. And then, Malede also joined because he was being trained as OBGYN resident at Black Lion, but primarily to work for them. So he fortunately finished that at that time, so he joined. So it was the five. But even before the three joined, myself and the original staff actually sat down together at a hotel off-site and started developing the curriculum.

So our small group of four sat down and drafted the first St. Paul OBGYN residency curriculum. So we took the Addis Ababa University curriculum, the curriculum at Gondar, the Jimma curriculum, and also, we took ideas from the University of Michigan. We took ideas and content from all those and drafted a competency-based curriculum, which was a new concept for residency training in Ethiopia. We sat down for three days or four to have the initial draft and then continue building on it.

T   Okay. But the curriculum was really written and developed by in-country Ethiopians—by the people in Ethiopia who were going to run the program?

L   Yes. Yes.

T   It wasn't imposed on you? It wasn't a foreign blueprint?

L   No. No, we had taken all those different curriculums and developed what would work best in our institution, but with contemporary aspects, like the competency basis.

T   So it was an Ethiopian planning team?

L   Yes. And the other support and input, after that, when this new group of doctors I mentioned joined, they also had the chance to review it before we actually launched it. So by the time it was launched, which was in 2012, it was all—it had input from many people. And then, during 2012, we recruited the first seven OBGYN residents. So it all happened—

T   So in 2012, you had seven residents. And then, have you had seven residents ever since then?

L   Oh, no. So the second one—it became fourteen.

T   So in 2013, it was fourteen residents?

L   In 2014, it was twenty-one, at least.

T   —and the duration of program was how many years?

L   Four years. Four years.

T   So by year three, you had forty-two residents in the training program?

L   Oh, yes.

T   So, so what's the, what's the—how many people do you currently intake now every year?

L   So there was a lot of interest from the minister of health to really increase that number. So St. Paul felt there was an effort to push us up, we got to a point that we didn't really want to increase because we wanted to maintain the quality. But there was this huge interest from the Ministry to increase our number. So the last recruit class was definitely, I know that it was thirty. So—but I think ultimately, it may not just continue to increase—

TI So at that same time, how many residents did they have a year at Black Lion? Were they taking thirty?

LR No, they would take around eighteen to twenty, around eighteen to twenty.

T So Black Lion was taking about twenty a year.

L Yes. Now they might have increased.

T And Jimma was taking about—

L Maybe not more than ten.

T And then Gondar was taking—

L —around ten. And now—so now, Black Lion—

T Their faculty has gone down too, really, with attrition, some to St. Paul's, hasn't it?

L Um, it had—it had gone down at some point, but now they have recruited new faculty who graduated from the residency, so they have now, new young people.

T But it didn't take long for St. Paul to become the largest training program in the country, right?

L Yes. It's very large now. And there has been a big increase in the number of faculty, even though it had five staff initially, then it continued to grow. And then, before the first group graduated in July 2016, that's when the first group graduated. Yeah, July 2016, and first OBGYN residents graduated, the seven. So before they graduated we had around sixteen OBGYN faculty.

T Sixteen faculty! And now, now there have been subspecialty training and you've got subspecialists and everything?

L Yes. The first group graduated in 2016, so—but the first fellowship was maternal-fetal medicine in 2017. So—

T So it started around the same time as the residency graduation, huh? And there are three fellows a year? How many a year?

L No, two, two a year.

T Two per year, for three years?

L Yes.

T And then...?

L Yes, and then family planning and REI [reproductive endocrinology and infertility]. Yeah.

T So OBGYN started in 2012. Pretty soon, there were other residencies that started, right?

L Yes. Yes.

T So emergency medicine was one?

L No. No. Emergency medicine started very late. So, so it continued. So then I continued reaching out to different people in the departments, here in St. Paul Millennial Hospital and Medical School [sic], and then the next one to start was surgery. General surgery.

T About 2014 do you think?

L A little later, I think. Following that, internal medicine.

T Okay. And then pediatrics?

L And then radiology started. It almost started the same time pediatrics started. So now, the programs are partnering with University of Michigan. And they even have fellowship programs in pediatrics, that they are really supported from Ann Arbor. And then ophthalmology. Ophthalmology and anesthesiology.

T And then, the kidney transplant program was another big piece.

L Oh, that's another big piece. Yes. That's another big piece.

T Which I think the first kidney transplants were done in—

L September 2015.

T I was just talking to Jeff Punch [transplant surgeon from Michigan] the other day. I think they've done forty now or something like that.

L Almost around forty, yeah. Yeah. The—they almost go every month too, and in one trip, they would do at least three to four transplants, and the transplant surgery is also—it includes also a transplant fellowship. So there are four fellows being trained by Jeff. So hopefully by—

T Are they graduates of the surgery program, do you think?

L No, they are—they used to be faculty at the—in the surgery department. The surgery program is about to graduate its first residents.

T Okay.

L So but these are faculty in the surgery program. General surgeons in the former practice. Now they are fellows, yeah.

T But in the future, they will be training fellows?

L Yes.

T Do you think they're going to keep training fellows? Is that the plan? And how many transplant surgeons does Ethiopia need?

L Yeah. So it may not be a big—it may not continue to be a big training, but they will definitely continue to train.

T Why do you think St. Paul was so successful?

L Well, it—for multiple reasons. One is, when the partnership started, it's really as you stated earlier, it was not kind of imposing anything on us. It was up to us locally to try to figure out what we needed, what the Ministry wanted, what St. Paul wanted. So it was based on what was the pressing need of the institution and the country and our priorities. So it was based on that. And more so, the solutions came collaboratively with the—from the faculty and the, the people on the ground. So it [Michigan] was supporting what was there, [GPTP] was the model.

T Okay. That's an important part of the Ghana model, the local management and local control and local authority, which I think is unusual. Often, programs in the United States come in and they say this is—you know, they have funding. They're from an NGO. They have a contract they have to fulfill and complete in a certain time period. They have a certain, often a clear idea of what they want to do.

L Yes. Exactly.

T And here, this was really—I mean, your leadership mattered. Having you and having strong leaders, and I think the fact that it was a woman leading a program at a new institution that was conceived to focus on women's health—all those things helped, especially since, as you said, maternal mortality was a national priority, and a new children and women's hospital was being built on the St. Paul's site.

L Absolutely, yes. This would be a center—not only would it be an innovational medical school, but it would be a center for, kind of, children and women's health. So the leadership commitment from both the [medical] school and the Ministry of Health, that was—that played a critical role.

T   So—and the combination of female leadership plus maternal/child health has made it a little bit different.

L   Yes. Yes. Absolutely.

T   Because Black Lion had a reputation as an established, patriarchal, male-dominated place, right?

L   Yes. At some point, we were looking at St. Paul. And we had a much better number of women in leadership—department chairs and others. That was intentional. And the provost was really committed to academic growth and, and the other thing is, obviously, the obvious big piece is the commitment of faculty leadership training. She was to really become interested in this effort, not just people from Michigan to be involved. That was one big piece. She was getting people engaged in this program, but also more involvement with the academic mission on the ground in—at St. Paul, at the Ministry, and more students and faculty and residents. So that was one big piece.

T   So faculty, students, and people at the Ministry?

L   Yes. Yes. Another factor was the components included in the program, especially in the faculty development piece, where the faculty really felt that they owned the program and they were exposed with international visitors—when they came—when they come here to observe, it was not academic skills or knowledge that they would get, but they also get leadership development and kind of how the system is run in terms of academia and academic medical centers together. So they brought—that brought a lot of culture change. We—at St. Paul, there's a big, different culture of the academics and the less academic services: how faculty engage with their students, with their residents, how they mentor them is clearly quite different than the models we at least are trained in in Black Lion. People saw differences when they visited Michigan. So that played a big role, the faculty development really benefiting from faculty exchange when they were coming. Also, the U of M faculty going there, transplanting their skills. Learning differences in systems and processes was also very helpful.

T   So visiting Michigan to see how the clinical operations ran—
    and also how leadership training, leadership development was
    approached.

L   Development, yes. There was also an additional leadership training
    piece, both with faculty and students and residents, that was
    happening by, locally, a part of this program. But definitely, seeing
    how—when they have not just the clinical—how patients are treated,
    not just the clinical skills or the training, how knowledge—but how
    the proper approaches to patient flow, the patient care, how the
    patients are communicated with, how residents work together with
    nurses, with their faculty. So all of this, how residents are evaluated.
    So the whole process gave them a full picture. So let me tell you one
    very nice story that we always are proud of, is [that] in Ethiopia, in
    any medical school or any hospital, attendings did not stay in the
    hospital for the night calls.

T   Okay.

L   They are usually in their home, and they are called if needed and
    come in. But once they saw how things are practiced at Michigan and
    the impact this would have for the quality of care and for the training,
    they came back to St. Paul and decided that the faculty was going to
    start staying in the hospital when they were on duty.

T   So when did that start?

L   So it started maybe a year after the residency, maybe 2013. So we
    always at least have one faculty on the floor, so twenty-four-hour,
    both weekend and overnight.

T   So that was a paradigm shift, really.

L   It was a big paradigm shift. It has also spread to other training hospitals.
    I believe they were spreading word of the benefits, clinical faculty or
    consultants going to the other departments or other hospitals. It had
    literally impacted the quality of care and the quality of training for
    the residents and medical students because practically before this, as
    a resident, you're handling everything during the night. And you see
    a lot of complicated cases during the night. It so happens that the
    most—the most complicated cases happen in the night. And in my
    training, we had taken care of them mostly by ourselves because we
    didn't have that faculty supervision and support.

T   Yeah, and you made clinical mistakes and then dug your way out
    of them.

L   Yeah.

T   In the United States, the requirement for in-house faculty attendings
    started in the early 1980s. Before that, there were no in-house
    attendings. And the worst things happen at night, right?

L   Exactly.

T   And perforations and ruptured uteruses and all those things.

L   Oh, yeah. Absolutely.

TI And there was nobody there to help you.

L   Yeah, exactly. So this shift is going on very well.

T   And there's been a fairly good bilateral exchange, hasn't there? There's
    been about as many people from Michigan going there as Ethiopian
    faculty and residents in the opposite direction. There have been lots
    of Ethiopians who have come here.

L   Come—definitely. It's still going on.

T   And the faculty still comes here. The fellows have all come here and
    spent time.

L   Our fellows come here.

T   The oncology fellows, the maternal-fetal medicine fellows.

L   Absolutely. Yes.

T   So the bilateral exchange has been good.

L   Yeah, it has been good. And the other big piece is the research—on
    the research aspect also. Much of that started with Doctor Richard
    Adanu, who talked about research capacity building already on his
    very first trip to Ghana. Then he came and gave several short courses
    on research skills. So the research was—it was previously designed
    in a way that they would start at the last year of the residency. It had
    mostly been that way before. But then it started even from the Year 1,
    they're exposed to some research training and support. And they were
    doing projects. And another Michigan faculty, like Doctor Vanessa
    Dalton, had been instrumental in supporting that.

T   I remember that Professor Richard Adanu from Ghana was one of the
    first people to introduce research methods training.

L   Oh, yes. Especially for the faculty, so as part of the University of
    Michigan and St. Paul collaboration had emerged a collaboration with

the University of Ghana. So he comes almost every year, sometimes even twice per year to come and do faculty development trainings on research. So his support has been also instrumental.

T Example of South-South partnership—an important partnership because I think that Ghana and Ethiopia at least know each other, right?

L Yeah.

T They, they know that the other person is there, so they can call on them.

L Absolutely. Yeah.

T Any other important lessons?

L So yeah, I mean, definitely you can say this is a model, this academic collaboration definitely has made us more sustainable.

T That's what my book is about. It's about engaged, academic global health. And it's about sustainability and capacity building and all those things. Because you guys actually use the Charter to some extent, didn't you? You used Charter principles.

L Yes. Yes. The principles, yes. I think Ethiopia was ready for the program. And Ghana showed us a model of how to do things, right? We knew what worked and what didn't work. Absolutely. That would have an effect—

T St. Paul could train other new places to have residency programs.

L Yes. Actually, most of the programs have now started, and St. Paul's residency programs have continued to grow. So now there are, at least, I think, nine residency programs all over the country. And the other one thing I did forget, in teacher and faculty, training is important, so (Doctor) Balkachew was a residency director when the program started. And he, through the Michigan partnership, he was trained in the postgraduate school of CREOG Program director school.

So he took that training, and later on, one more person from Mekelle University was also trained. And they, last year, actually, they organized with Balkachew and one person from CREOG, they organized the training for all residency program directors all over the country, mostly OBGYN from all over the country, but for St. Paul's, even other program directors for the other residencies were included. So they were transferring that skill of running the program. So Balkachew's leadership is running a strong residency program, is also one of the strengths of the program, and the support he got from that training had impacted him.

T That's a good story too. Was the OBGYN medical student curriculum pretty well established before the residency was introduced? What impact was it on the medical school?

L Two key things about the medical school: One is the project that we have worked on integrating family planning, contraception, and abortion training into the medical school. Medical students in Ethiopia, what makes it different from the US is that they graduate—we graduate and work as general practitioners in rural practice. When we go to the district and rural areas all over the country, we are finding these general practitioners who include reproductive health services in their practice.

T So there was an introduction or enhancement of family planning and reproductive health curriculum?

L There was a gap in the curriculum, that necessary skills were not being included in teaching, especially in long-acting reversible contraceptive measures and abortion and postabortion techniques. That was one big change that was made through this collaboration, was [that] the curriculum was revised to incorporate a competency-based, skills-intensive training in family planning and abortion. And the other addition was to ensure that they had leadership training before they graduated. And that was through this curriculum, which included making sure that they had hands-on training in simulations and also clinical applications, that they have the clinical competency skills on those services. So both the leadership and this training have really helped them. We have seen the first graduates, after they went off to do work, after six months, an assessment was done on how they were practicing. And most of them were really engaged in the family planning and reproductive health services, even establishing services where there was no service when they were assigned and taking a lot of leadership roles in community education, outreach, and program building. Even as medical directors or other important local positions championing quality of care. So we've seen that the collaboration and the residency has also that kind of impact in the medical school curriculum.

T   I guess the other thing that may be equally important is that you had residents—you had quality residents who were teaching too, right?

L   Yes. I mean, they were seeing not just the faculty, but really the residents every day. Residents as teachers. There was some successful trainings, we are now working to make it actually integrated into the residency curriculum. To make our residents as teachers.

T   Great. Yeah, because I think when medical students see successful OBGYN residents, then they might think that's what they want to be, right?

L   Oh, yes. It is good recruitment.

T   Are the medical students at St. Paul about half women and half men?

L   Yeah. So that's one of the strengths of St. Paul is we try to assure that—and it has been around 40 percent woman or more in each class. In all years it is probably forty-sixty female. And we are hoping it will grow more.

T   Yeah. Almost everywhere in the world, the smartest students are girls.

L   Well, that's a big change. When I was a medical student, it was less than 10 percent.

T   So Ethiopia was late to the gender shift.

L   Yes. Yes.

T   And do you think that now, [the] number going into OBGYN, is it about fifty-fifty?

L   Not yet. One thing is the overall number of physicians graduating. Woman physicians graduating are overall lower than men, but the percentage of women joining OBGYN residency is also lower.

T   Why do you think that is?

L   We are doing a project trying to study now why are women not joining OBGYN. And I think mostly it's because of the quality of life; it demands a lot.

T   So what do most graduating women physicians in Ethiopia do?

L   A lot of them do pediatrics or radiology. I've seen more women also do internal medicine. They would tend to do non-surgical specialties.

T   Well, that's a challenge everywhere. That's certainly a challenge in Ghana. Thanks for a great discussion.

Lessons Learned

Innovation is reproducible.

Local management and control is foundational.

South-South collaboration works.

Faculty development in education and research builds academic capacity.

Teaching residents to teach is important for development and recruitment.

Gender equity needs to be an intentional goal in medical education and academic medicine at every level.

Chapter 11

The Opportunities, Roles, and Responsibilities of Academic Institutions

A discussion of academic global health engagement is timely because there is so much demand. Up to 60 percent of current US medical students are interested in a global experience. A burgeoning number of undergraduate students across multiple disciplines and schools are also interested in global and international issues. Many of them are engaging in service-learning trips (see Chapter 6) and in joining various NGOs, and even founding them. Many undergraduates seek global opportunities after graduation with the Peace Corps or NGOs. Medical residents in training and practicing physicians both young and older seek involvement in global health opportunities and activities. Given this demand by students, universities must think intentionally and seriously about how, and whether, they are going to provide these opportunities. This may include coursework, academic minors and majors, and transnational and international programs for learners, faculty, and alumni.

Universities, as one of the great institutions of Western civilization, can engage, teach, train, implement, innovate, and sustain. In many high-income countries, universities have substantial independence from governments and other external agents. The suggestion that universities can be a nexus for global partnerships and share their academic values is one whose time has come. The students and learners at universities include undergraduates, graduate students, professionals in the medical school and in other healing arts schools, residents, postdoctoral fellows, medical specialists, medical subspecialists, and simply lifelong learners who are interested to thoughtfully develop in obtaining medical education. Meeting the needs of such a large and disparate group will be challenging.

Who Are Our "Global" Students/Learners?

- Undergraduate
- Graduate
- Professional (medical school)
- Interprofessional opportunities (medicine, nursing, public health, dentistry, engineering)
- Residency/postdoctoral
- Medical specialist
- Medical subspecialist
- Lifelong learner/continuing medical education

This educational context provides a framework for responsible institutions to develop programs that are both ethical and sustainable. Universities should ensure that they and their academic partners have established programs, that students can engage in these programs safely, and that they have appropriate supervision by faculty. Institutions may find that partnering with other institutions might allow them to broaden and deepen the quality of the programs among institutions, as one institution cannot "do it all," and sharing high-quality programs is an excellent approach. The Charter compact, designed for global partnership, probably would be an appropriate framework between partnering institutions within countries and local regions.

Global academic programs should be curriculum-based milestones and competencies that are measured in a rigorous, contemporary fashion. If faculty at all participating schools are engaged, the supervision of students can occur at any school, especially if curriculum, milestones, and competencies are shared among the faculty. Each student should expect to have evaluation and feedback, and this should occur at least midway through the experience and again at the end. The possibility of academic credit should be considered. If the learners are medical students who do this as their clinical or fourth-year electives, there should be academic evaluations, but participating medical residents will need competency-based clinical evaluations and evaluation based on Accreditation Council for Graduate Medical Education (ACGME) milestones. There can be an opportunity for participation in research, again possibly for credit, as appropriate, and/or the possibility of presentations or publications. Other students may pay for the service-learning experience and receive experiential credit, often required for professional school or employment applications, rather than academic credit. These students, at whatever level, should have some type of a viable academic or private-sector pathway for advancement or employment that is explicit and realistic when they enter a global pathway program. Students should demand that these experiences be constructed in ways that are ethical, represent values of both social justice and equity, and are shared between the learner and their institution. Students should assess and consider the importance of having their global experience be in the context of sustained partnerships and programs, both reflecting respectful institutional principles, and because the learners may often develop their own lifelong partnerships and relationships that will be meaningful and important for their future. Institutional relationships should always remain self-aware, mutually honest, and adhere to the Charter principles as described (Chapter 8).

What Students Should Expect

ESTABLISHED PROGRAMS

SAFETY

SUPERVISION

CURRICULUM

EVALUATION AND FEEDBACK

ACADEMIC CREDIT

VIABLE ACADEMIC (OR OTHER SECTOR) CAREER
PATHWAY

What Students Should Demand

ETHICAL (BILATERAL)

SUSTAINABLE

TRANSPARENCY

"CHARTER" PRINCIPLES

There are numerous advantages to institutions who do this well and right. Global programs can serve to recruit students at all levels. As we have seen, they can engender collaborative research across all domains including the humanities, social sciences, and basic and medical sciences. Collaboration and exchanges of faculty can encourage transnational, interdisciplinary, and transdisciplinary scholarship. Global partnerships can feed the "publish or perish" monster for all concerned. These possibilities have been embraced by the recent presidents of the University of Michigan, who have both spoken about the academic opportunities of global partnerships and of the need to enter them equitably and honorably.

In 2008 Mary Sue Coleman, president of the University of Michigan, decided to personally demonstrate the University's commitment to expanding its global programs by initiating an international tour. Her staff reviewed faculty and school engagement in global education and discussed that there were substantial programs extant in Ghana, including Ray Silverman in Museum Studies, and our own extensive medical initiatives (Silverman 2015; Silverman et al., 2021.

Plans for the tour were announced, and the first port of call for the presidential delegation was announced as Ghana.

A few weeks before her planned visit I received a call from her office asking what type of "swag" she could take that would be well received. Note pads and pens were suggested. After some thought about issues like cost, uniqueness, and something that would be broadly welcomed, I recommended lapel pins with the University of Michigan "block M" flag and the flag of Ghana. The UM alumni association had been distributing pins combining the American flag with the university's "block M" flag (maize on blue), and I knew they had been widely distributed and popular. The "MichiGhana" pins were ordered and were incredibly well received. They were unique and "on brand." President Coleman could not have had a gift that was more warmly received by students, faculty, and even the minister of education. By the end of the trip our partners in Ghana, and the Michigan faculty and staff, were all wearing MichiGhana pins. They continue to be produced and given to visiting students, residents, and faculty from Ghana and are worn by Michigan students and faculty who go to Ghana. They are striking statement pieces are very low cost. They became so popular and well-recognized that programs in Ethiopia, Brazil, and China all created their own Michigan flag lapel pins (jewelry!) with their national flags. Of course, Ghana students also stock up on Michigan T shirts and sweatshirts, usually printed with "Michigan Medical School." Walking around Ghana campuses today, it is not surprising to see young people in Michigan Medical School T shirts and MichiGhana pins. It was and remains great marketing and branding.

Several UM faculty, including several involved with the GPTP, went ahead to prepare a program and welcome the president upon her arrival. Waiting for the arrival of President Mary Sue Coleman in the VIP lounge of Kotoko Airport in Accra was clear evidence that the University of Michigan leadership might be supportive of the concept of platforms and long-term partnership. The lounge was air-conditioned but had large, handmade wooden chairs and couches covered with heavy, warm material and heavily carpeted floors. How different from my outdoor entrance and arrivals in 1986, although I had since discovered that here had been, and still existed, this isolated VIP reception room for governmental dignitaries.

Mary Sue Coleman met with the leaders of KNUST and KATH and other important functionaries and participated in productive, candid meetings. The substantive health science discussions between central administration and its leaders were just starting at KATH when Mary Sue Coleman went to meet with the Asantehene, the paramount king of the Ashanti Region. As much as I had dreamed of an audience at Manhyia Palace (the Asantehene's palace), the continuing discussions at the health sciences campus needed the catalyst of my presence.

Later, President Coleman had a very important meeting with KNUST Vice-Chancellor K. K. Adarkwa. (Vice-chancellor is the university president equivalent in the British system; chancellor of Ghana universities is an honorary position given to luminaries such as Kofi Annan at the University of Ghana and the Asantehene at KNUST.)

She asked me to accompany her to the meeting, then, when I held back, asked me to accompany her into the vice-chancellor's office, which occupied an office on a top floor of a building that dominated the campus, located on top of a hill that was central to the campus. It commanded a breathtaking view of the campus below and the colorfully painted houses and gardens of the city beyond: Kumasi is known as the "garden city." President Coleman walked in, preceded by the university "protocol officer." The vice-chancellor was an imposing man who stood behind his desk, his own private view across the campus and the city was afforded through the window behind him. The protocol officer formally intoned: "Vice-Chancellor, I present President Mary Sue Coleman, the president of the Michigan State University." In that instant, President Coleman looked at me and I looked at her, and the same message passed silently between us: should we correct the introduction? Of course, the University of Michigan and Michigan State University are two different, very strongly competitive interstate institutions. The athletic and academic rivalries and competition between the schools were legend, and often "divided" families, including allegiances in my own. In that instant, the silent decision that mutually passed between us was to just "let it go" as Vice-Chancellor (V-C) Adarkwa came around his desk to greet President Coleman. As he put out his hand, however, the first words of out the V-C's mouth were: "No, no, she is the President of the University of Michigan, not Michigan State University. The University of Michigan is maize and blue, and Michigan State is green and white! The University of Michigan is in Ann Arbor and Michigan State University is in East Lansing. I know, I did my PhD in Urban Planning at Michigan State. I spent many pleasant years in East Lansing, but I have visited Ann Arbor! I loved my time in Michigan!" The world suddenly became very small. Another look flashed between President Coleman and me—"You can't make this up!"—and she went on to have a pleasant discussion, president to vice-chancellor, about the potential for collaboration between their two universities, with the clear understanding that international interactions and common interests were demonstrably long-standing, common, and frequent. V-C Adarkwa appreciated the "MichiGhana" lapel flags President Coleman gave him, even more so since he recognized the maize and blue "block M" from his own graduate student days. For me this was just one of hundreds of propitious, serendipitous, but meaningful "moments" of my own Ghana experience.

Back in Accra, there was a lovely reception hosted by Mary Sue Coleman at the Kofi Annan International Peacekeeping Training Centre in Teshie on the Tema Road. The Family Health Hospital already existed, but it would later grow into a complex with a nursing school and then a medical school. It was a very collegial and warm reception, and Mary Sue Coleman was surrounded by students. She gave several speeches in Accra attended by academics, members of Parliament, and representatives from the Ministry of Health and the Ministry of Education. MichiGhana pins were widely distributed. All her speeches were about academics and academic partnership. Her first global and African trip started in Ghana, just as Barack Obama would later start his introductory trip to Africa with a stop in Ghana. She then traveled to South Africa and then the Middle East. After her trip, it was clear that Michigan intended to advance its engagement in global education.

She later made an important trip to China. The University of Michigan now had a presidential mandate to expand its global footprint and continue on a path of long-term academic partnership.

Soon after her return from Africa, Mary Sue Coleman spoke about Michigan's global engagement, the Ghana project, and my role in it, at the 2008 University-wide Honors Convocation:

> Just a few days ago I returned from leading a delegation of university faculty to Ghana and South Africa, and during those travels I was eyewitness to communities and universities that do not enjoy all the advancements we take for granted in our every-day lives.
>
> We think nothing of going into one of our library buildings, always expecting to find whatever reference we seek, because our collections (and our progress in digitization) are so vast. We would be dismayed not to have access to the very latest in scientific instruments, or appropriate laboratory space for almost any type of experiment we could imagine. But these are luxuries that are not often found in other parts of the world, including areas of Africa.
>
> This is a region of the world rich in people, culture, and history, but poor in technology. Yet what is lacking in technological wizardry is overshadowed by the commitment of individuals to improve the health and well-being of Ghanaians and South Africans.
>
> We saw that in Dr. Timothy Johnson, the chair of our Department of Obstetrics and Gynecology and a long-time visitor to Ghana. Dr. Johnson is a familiar face in West Africa, having spent more than 20 years training Ghanaian doctors who are committed to furthering their education and practicing medicine in their communities.
>
> In fact, he is received like a rock star because of his good deeds. It was really quite remarkable to witness the reception he encounters. Dr. Johnson is beloved in Ghana because he is dedicated to saving the lives of mothers-to-be. Maternal mortality rates in Ghana are among the highest in the world, and Dr. Johnson's training is designed to reduce pregnancy-related deaths among women by equipping Ghanaian physicians with the tools they need.

Just as important as providing this high-quality training is that it is conducted in Ghana. This is not a case of "come to America because we know what is best for you." Ghanaian doctors in this program tell us they want to practice medicine in their homeland, and providing this training locally allows them to make the life-saving contributions they envisioned when they decided to become doctors.

The results are astounding: Sixty-two physicians have trained in the program, and all but one has stayed in Ghana to practice medicine. That's more than five dozen doctors prepared to help women and their babies through the ordeal of childbirth, often in rural settings far removed from today's technologies.

This collaborative training program is a win-win for doctors and the patients they serve. I met a number of medical students currently enrolled in the program and their pride in what they could do for their country was palpable. It is particularly rewarding when you learn that nationwide, 60 percent of medical specialists who were trained in Ghana (in non-U-M programs) leave to practice in other countries.

This is the power of individuals to launch a revolution—to think beyond themselves to spark a revolution of life-saving health care that will resonate for generations.

(Website accessed 11/7/2020)

When he succeeded Mary Sue Coleman as President, Mark Schlissel, an academic physician and basic science researcher, endorsed President Coleman's commitment to global partnership and endorsed fair principles of global academic partnership in a piece he wrote for the *Times Higher Education*, a British publication. He recognized the blueprint presented by the Ghana program and directly addressed many of the key features of the Charter as critical features of equitable and mutually beneficial academic partnerships. He has been particularly interested and personally involved in enhancing UM engagement in China, especially Shanghai Jiao Tong University and Beijing University.

Schlissel Comments from *Times Higher Education*, March 2015

Trust exercises
March 11, 2015
Mark Schlissel comments:

Michigan's long-term commitment in West and East Africa provides a rich model for symbiotic global education, argues Mark S. Schlissel.

Research universities have enormous potential to deliver meaningful change in areas of the world facing severe resource challenges. Global education that focuses on mutual benefits among partners is the key that can unlock that potential.

When physician Tim Johnson first travelled to Ghana in 1986, the West African nation had just five obstetricians serving a population of 12 million. While many Ghanaians trained in medicine abroad, few came back to work in their home country.

Three years later, Johnson led the University of Michigan in a partnership with medical schools in Ghana that would address two major challenges for the country: training Ghanaian physicians at home and combating high rates of maternal mortality.

Retaining trained healthcare providers in developing countries is a primary factor in improving health outcomes and achieving UN Millennium Development Goals to improve maternal health and reduce child mortality.

Under the programme established by the Michigan-Ghana collaboration, 142 physicians have been trained and 141 are still in the country.

The blueprint established by Johnson, now chair of the department of obstetrics and gynaecology at Michigan, led to a formal charter in 2009 between Ghana and Michigan that outlines both sides' common responsibilities to clinical service, research and education.

Since then, additional projects have taken off in the country. Built on a foundation of trust and reciprocity, these projects involve scholars and students from disciplines including engineering, public health, history, and art and design. This summer, 20 Michigan undergraduates will live with 20 local students in Kumasi, Ghana. Together they will learn entrepreneurship and how to assess technology needs.

The success in Ghana is an example of Michigan's approach to global education. It is deeply rooted in the university's culture and public ethos, which seeks to co-create mutual opportunities for its students and academics with people and communities abroad.

Michigan's approach begins with collaboration. Academics develop relationships with local colleagues in areas such as education, industry and government, with the aim of fostering long-term benefits for both sides. Together the partners examine problems from the local point of view and work to craft locally driven solutions. It is about being partners, not competitors. These collaborations allow for increases in capacity, as starting "small" gives successful ideas room to grow.

The final part of the Michigan approach is to leverage the lessons learned from the collaborations and capacity building into initiatives that cross disciplines, regions and even international borders. The result is a lasting contribution that inspires more collaboration.

Senait Fisseha, professor of obstetrics and gynaecology at Michigan, is using this approach in Ethiopia to address a maternal mortality rate that is among the highest in the world.

Fisseha was born in Ethiopia and met Johnson during her residency at Michigan. Her passion was to work in her native country: at Johnson's recommendation, she began building relationships with academics, health professionals and government officials there.

Her meetings with the Ethiopian health minister in 2011 led to a partnership between Michigan and St Paul's Hospital Millennium Medical College, based in the capital city of Addis Ababa.

The "Ghana model" had inspired action in a nation on the other side of the continent.

The collaboration initially resulted in a programme to train physicians—with those instructed in Ghana helping to launch the Ethiopian programme—but because of Michigan's long history in Africa, the seeds for something bigger had already been sown.

Michigan students at all levels and staff from disciplines across the full campus are involved. Projects include setting up a computer lab at the Addis Ababa Institute of Technology to give Ethiopian students access to equipment needed for education in technology; and academics are exploring providing Amharic language instruction for Michigan students in Ethiopia.

Nearly 50 investigators from 15 Michigan Medical School departments are now involved in Ethiopia. Student volunteers from the university are engaging in valuable experiential learning under an Ethiopian health ministry programme that provides exposure to medical conditions that are rare in the US.

Fisseha recently received a $25 million (£16.4 million) grant that will allow her to create a centre for reproductive health training in her home country. It will increase the number of health professionals in Africa who can provide life-saving reproductive healthcare, especially to women from poor backgrounds.

Michigan's approach to global education—collaboration, capacity building and leveraging, all driven by mutual benefits—is working all over the world, with programmes developed on six continents. To help build further momentum, the university has expanded its reach through websites translated into Hindi, Mandarin, Portuguese and Spanish.

Universities have the ability to make sustainable, decades-long commitments in nations where there are no short-term solutions. And with the right approach, we can provide learning opportunities and partnerships that provide immense value around the world and here in Ann Arbor.

Mark S. Schlissel
President, University of Michigan

These comments were particularly meaningful to me, coming from Mark Schlissel. I knew he had received his MD and PhD from Johns Hopkins during the time I was on the faculty there. When we met for the first time, with a twinkle in his eye, he said, as we shook hands: "You won't remember me, but when I was a third-year student I did my first delivery, and you were the supervising faculty." Medical students never forget their first delivery; it may be the most highly anticipated rite of passage during a medical education. After close to twenty thousand deliveries in my career, I certainly don't remember many medical students that I have shared that experience with, but I am forever grateful for the opportunity to have been a bedside obstetrician to assist so many women and families hopefully achieve safe motherhood.

A specific and attractive example of the kind of successful undergraduate experiences that can be achieved in global engagement and global health is Yaera Spraggins who, as a freshman at the University of Michigan, responded to an opportunity to help with research on the experience of UM medical students in Ghana and other global clinical rotations, which was described in a University publication:

Yaera Spraggins, Recently Published Undergraduate Research Opportunity Program (UROP) Alumni

What made you choose UROP?
This may sound cliche but I chose UROP for the research experience. I was oblivious to what research really entailed. I always thought of it as surfing through the internet in search of the meaning of a word or going to the laboratory in your lab coat to conduct chemical reactions. But through UROP, I have learned that research comprises of all these and more. Now, I know how to conduct research effectively to yield desired results, as well as analyzing data and finding common trends in specific research.

What UROP Program(s) were you a part of?
The First-Year Traditional UROP 2019–2020

Have you kept in contact with your research mentor?
Yes! I was able to reach out to my mentor beginning of this semester.

How did your UROP experience shape or inform the next steps you took in your academic and professional journey?
With the experience I have gained from UROP and especially working for my mentor, I plan to possibly minor in Women's and Gender

studies. My research project reviewed reflections by the University of Michigan medical students who had completed rotations in hospitals in Ghana. Most of these students rotated in the Obstetrics and Gynecology Department, and expressed that they appreciate the exposure to different health populations, the hands-on surgical experience, and building cross-cultural relationships. They also shared that there is work that still needs to be done in improving the general health of women and I would love to be apart of that team, thus goal to attain this minor.

What drew you to the research project you worked on?

What drew me to the research project was its connection to my origins. I was born and raised in Ghana, West Africa, and was ecstatic to find that there was such a project led by a brilliant and wonderful individuals who are familiar with the country and spend most of their time there. It was not surprising that I immediately applied for the project upon realizing how honored I would be working for the betterment of my people.

What was the most exciting part of the project?

The project focused on the student exchange partnership that the University of Michigan has with major universities in Ghana, so students had the opportunity to go to Ghana and some students were able to come to this university as well. In November last year, 4 Ghanaian medical students came to the US and although I did not get to know them personally, I enjoyed meeting them. Not only did we have meaningful conversations about the rotations they were planning to do and how impactful it would be, they brought back stories from home that I missed dearly. Hopefully, when I go back home, I would be able to reconnect with them!

What are some recent publications or accomplishments that you are proud of?

Embedding international medical student electives within a 30-year partnership: the Ghana-Michigan collaborationhttps://bmcmededuc. biomedcentral.com/articles/10.1186/s12909-020-02093-6

What advice would you give to a current UROP student?

Be patient with the project search, you will definitely get into a project that you would hopefully love! I say this because it took me some time to get myself the project I worked on. I applied for about 10 projects and was called back for 2 interviews, all of which I got rejected. I began contemplating whether to quit the program and reapply my sophomore year because it was in the middle of October and I did not know if I would get a project or not. However, my peer facilitator recommended not to do so and I am glad I listened to her because the last project I applied to was the one I got accepted! The application process may be tedious but once you get your hands on that project, you would appreciate the time you waited patiently for it.

(Undergraduate Research Opportunity Program, 2020)

As we have discussed, research is a great opportunity for learner engagement that academic institutions almost uniquely can offer. We saw that demonstrated at the undergraduate level with Emma Lawrence, and now in the specific context of academic priorities with Yaera Spraggins. Doing research for medical students informs them about the source and basis of evidence-based practice in way that reading a book would never do. Undergraduate students can test whether a science and/or a medical future is for them. All are better able to review the literature, and many learn identify those studies that show real promise or are paradigm shifting and are able to use clinical research, translational research, or basic science research to change their future practice in important ways.

Experience for all level of learners is what has been called the "implicit curriculum"—often behavioral or attitudinal changes. Between the US students going to Ghana and Ghana students going to the United States, we have collected a fair amount of data, and in past experiences the students from Ghana learn about patient care, informed consent, and patients getting a complete discussion of their disease rather than a patriarchal "talking-down" model that they have seen before. Introduction to technology is also important. Several papers from our group have demonstrated the kinds of benefits that students have experienced (Abedini et al., 2014, 2015; Danso-Bamfo et al., 2017; Lawrence et al., 2020).

One of the issues that must be talked about is the generational differences we are seeing in our learners. Gen X and especially millennials
tend to approach life in a different way, and I believe that in the contemporary environment, universities need to be much more engaged with
student learners and listen to and act on student learners' feedback.
They need to be responsive to learner suggestions and they need to
be able to change their programs in a rapid way using lessons learned
from both their global partners and student learners. Often students
have excellent ideas for changes that can occur in curriculum, program
structure, institutional practices, and instructor delivery. Our current
students can be engaged as partners in their learning process and
develop leadership roles as they pursue their educational goals. This
is now recognized as part of the lifelong paradigm of academic medicine, where the traditional three-legged stool—clinical care, teaching,
and research—is beginning to recognize the importance of a fourth
leg: leadership, advocacy, and activism. This applies now to learners at
all levels, who as part of their education can receive and benefit from
both explicit and implicit education on leadership principles. Global
programs are a great way to build leadership confidence and competency for participating learners.

What Universities Need to Do in the New Millennium When Dealing with Gen Xers and Millennials

- Listen to/act on student (learner) feedback.
- Be responsive to student (learner) suggestions.
- CHANGE using lessons learned from partners and students (learners).

What Universities Can Change Using Lessons Learned and Feedback from Partners and Students (Learners)

- Curriculum
- Programs
- Institutional practices and structures
- Students (learners) as engaged partners and (future) leaders

Students can themselves work with institutions to build endowments, develop charters, and participate in evaluations and outcome metrics. In fact, the process of funding and developing programs that have a strong curriculum, that are developmentally appropriate and ethically grounded, makes participation a "teachable moment" and part of the learning experience.

Perhaps rather than raising money for their own NGOs and individual projects, they can be part of university fundraising for global programs and endowments. Perhaps a discussion of financial considerations will also provide a useful teachable experience: finances are always foundational. Even for universities it is ultimately true that "no money, no mission." With all the advantages of university structure and sustainability, it must be said that university finance can be byzantine and challenging. One lesson from my many years in academic medicine is that the funds flow process and budgeting are continuously changing, in fact often yearly, making financial planning and projections different. For example, I have seen even such basic financing principles as cash versus accrual accounting change from year to year in departments and medical schools. Knowing my strengths and weaknesses—and this is an important message for career planning and leadership—I have always selected someone with an MBA as my senior administrative partner. I have come to recognize that I went into clinical medicine and academics because of clinical strengths, research inclinations, and a commitment to teaching. I was not good at accounting and economics and did not want to do the work of an MBA or get an MBA, so I found partners to cover those important interests.

Academic medical centers have long taken advantage of "indirect costs," which are a common addition to NIH grants used to defray administrative and structural overhead (Appendix 6). Universities have to hire secretarial support, but also mow the lawns, keep the lights on, and provide security, among many other things. In the United States these costs have been covered by generous indirect costs, often 50 percent or more that are automatically added to and paid on many NIH grants. These allow universities and their schools and colleges, notably schools of medicine and clinical departments, to cover administrative overhead. Each university handles disbursement of these funds differently, with some or all kept centrally, distributed to schools, departments, or principal investigators as incentives to get and keep grants. These indirect costs have been a major source of funding and success for US academic medical centers (AMCs) for decades.

Challenges come with grants from foundations and for-profit entities such as pharmaceutical companies and device manufacturers, who do not want to pay a 50 percent premium over and above the costs of the program or research they want to fund at an AMC. They are willing to pay some percentage for administrative costs of the researchers, often 10 to 15 percent, but the research must be aware of the financial flow of their organization. Often there are taxes on these grants, for example a provost's tax of 15 percent to support central university activities, or a dean's tax of 10 to 12 percent to support the medical school or college involved. If the grant is only paying 10 percent to support the researcher's administrative costs not directly paid by the grant (possibly copy-making, rent, secretarial support), then the grantee may end up having to find the equivalent of 25 percent of the grant from other sources to "have the privilege" of receiving the grant. Institutions often have perverse disincentives that need to be constantly considered in funding, including funding for a global health initiative.

As an example, for many years, my medical school administration required a minimum of 12 percent indirect payment to them on any grant or contract. An important and popular training program mechanism to train and fund junior faculty members was the so-called K-grant mechanism. These grants that supported early career trainees, including the academic training and research, only provided 8 percent for indirect costs. If the OBGYN department wanted to support trainees with the program, it had to pay 4 percent from other department resources or funds to add to the 8 percent to make the required 12 percent payment to the school, leaving no administrative overhead or discretionary dollars for the department. Given the importance of such training programs to the careers of young faculty, and therefore the future department, clinical revenues were often used (diverted from other uses) to pay this tax, but it required the conscious assent of the department leadership to make this commitment and investment. The incentives and disincentives of each university are different and must be understood.

When dealing with grants and contracts for global health work, the issues of taxes and funds flow must be carefully understood and considered. If the university and school taxes are not considered when the contracts are made, the recipients might find themselves having to find sources of funds to pay for shortfalls required to fulfill the deliverables of the contract. This is no doubt why many foundations end up contracting with NGOs, which do not have the same requirements for indirect cost support, indirect cost recovery, and complicated administrative taxation. It is also a reason why many projects, grants, and contracts that are initially housed in academic departments and institutions end up "spinning off" into academically affiliated but no longer academic-based NGOs. One of the things that academic faculty and students involved with global health will need to do is renegotiate and reframe the cost structure for doing global health work in academic institutions (see what students need to do in global health, Chapter 6).

Failure of academic institutions to attend to this funds flow issue with extramural grants and contracts supporting global health will stifle institutional engagement and success, and institutions who purport to support global health opportunities for students, other learners, and faculty have a responsibility to get this right, rather than offering only disincentives and, even worse, perverse incentives to engage in global health work.

Universities also must understand that educational programs and research programs are not money earners, unlike clinical departments and hospitals that have long provided much of the support for AMCs. Education must be paid for by tuition, state or institutional funds, grants and contracts, or excess clinical revenues. The same goes for research. I don't know of anywhere where educational revenues, whatever the source, or research revenues, whatever the source, are adequate and sufficient to support the modern AMC or university. The addition of global health initiatives will need the same attention to support and resources to achieve the word we have used repeatedly in the context of global health: sustainability.

Universities who become global partners will find that the return on the investment of people, money, and time will be very positive. The major lesson for me is that I have gained much more from my global engagement and projects than I feel I have given in these relationships. People always say, "Thank you so much for the work you have done in Ghana," but, as I have said before, the insights I have had on relationships between academics and public health, leadership opportunities, grant management opportunities, research opportunities, and the opportunity to nurture students from different cultures as medical students, residents, and fellows have all been much more impactful on me than any contributions I think I have made in the global space. Working in low-income countries without some of the previous infrastructure, policies, and processes in the United States allows one to think about clinical redesign in a way that would otherwise not be as innovative and flexible. These experiences have been a learning and growing experience for me, and I have observed, as both presidents have spoken about, that the same applies to universities. In global partnerships, in addition to thinking strategically, opportunistically, and ethically, what one learns experientially may apply to other partnerships, either global or domestic. Much of my advocacy and activism for domestic issues, and much of my passion for global health, comes from what I have learned in and from Ghana.

What is the goal of universities and colleges in developing an ethical and sustainable portfolio of offerings in the global space? It is ultimately to develop global citizens and develop programmatic offerings and research initiatives that support their mission to advance the lives of these global citizens. Training students in their professions and encouraging them to engage the world, especially as advocates and activists, is one aspiration consistent with experiences in the global space. Students have long been advocates and activists. What should these student learners do? They should advocate that universities offer global opportunities that are pedagogically serious and ethically constructed.

This means universities need to provide the programs that meet learner needs and to use university funds or raise the money through philanthropy to support this type of important global work. Students need to be advocates for this. Student voices can and should hold their institutions to programmatic standards that are transparent and fair to all concerned.

How to Think about Academic Global Health within a Human Rights and Sustainable Development Goals (SDG) Framework

- TRATEGICALLY
- OPPORTUNISTICALLY
- ETHICALLY

HEALTH AS A HUMAN RIGHT IS A DISRUPTIVE AND TRANSFORMATIVE IDEA

The global academic engagement proposed in this model is fundamentally disruptive and radical, but it can be transformative and sustainable and lead to progressive changes in academic partnerships. These partnerships are like a laboratory, a laboratory in the model of implementation science to introduce best practices, whether they are pedagogic or medical. Doing experiments within this partnership allows for testing of educational and clinical policies and practice. It allows for modification and adaptability, and with the resultant changes the new and developing programs can become a paradigm for future programs and interventions. The reminder that publication is important for replication to occur is obviously a personal mantra, and the secondary benefit of academic achievement and recognition for the authors is an advantageous bonus. This allows one to think about academic global health and human rights in a sustainable fashion. The sustainable goals follow the life development goals and, using the human rights framework and SDG framework (see table), allows one to set priorities. It remains an unfortunate fact that health as a human right remains a disruptive and transformative idea.

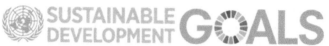
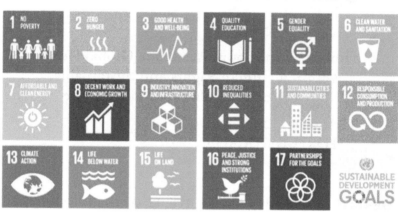

Lessons Learned

Institutions have ethical responsibilities to their students and global partners.

Student must expect programs that are, at a minimum, safe, established, supervised, and academically credible.

Students must hold institutions accountable for transparent, mutually beneficial global partnerships.

CHAPTER 12

"The Dream Goes On…": The Development of Academic and Individual Global Leaders and Leadership

At one of the events marking a GPTP success, perhaps when the first woman graduate of the program was receiving her certificate of completion from the hands of the then civilian president of Ghana, Flight Lieutenant Jerry Rawlings (he of the PNDC and Osu Castle adventure of 1986), I was sitting next to Doctor J. B. Wilson, and he said to me: "The dream goes on." Since then, at numerous celebrations in Ghana we have savored the moment with each other and said, sometimes in a whisper, sometimes out loud, and sometimes in a speech: "The dream goes on." This reflects the success story I have told so far, the unexpected ways it has expanded and influenced individuals, institutions, and countries, and the knowledge that it will continue to do so in unknowable ways for the foreseeable future. The opportunities for clinical teaching; undergraduate, medical student, resident, and fellow teaching; faculty development; research across multiple domains; implementation science and a partnership with colleagues developing implementation engineering and design science; and finally, the development of numerous clinical programs in OBGYN and numerous other specialty disciplines in Ghana, and then in Ethiopia—all demonstrate a broad impact of the GPTP. The Charter document presents generalizable principles to inform global health partnerships, and Ethiopia shows how those principles can be used by other institutions to develop programs and projects that replicate the successes in Ghana. These principles, fundamentally ethical principles, go beyond nonmaleficence and beneficence, and although mutual benefit is one of the requirements for successful partnership, there are many others that must be attended to in order to ensure successful and sustainable long-term global partnerships.

Others have recognized this:

> You have to make sure that the global partnership is bidirectional and that the needs of the people in the country you're working with are getting put in front of yours. I think we, as researchers here in Michigan, can craft our research questions to go along with those needs and priorities. At U-M, there are such amazing opportunities for medical students to go abroad, and on the flipside, there are such ideal examples of how sustainable global collaborations can be made. That's one of the strengths that globally sets us apart at the global level. We have leaders that insist right out of the gate that everything we do has to be bidirectional, has to be long-term. These aren't "one-and-done" projects—let's make sure that we're making a difference.
>
> Jason Bell, MD, MPH, MS, assistant professor of
> obstetrics and gynecology, associate director of the
> UM Medical School Global Health and Disparities
> Path of Excellence (Michigan Medicine, 2016)

Sujal Parikh was a UM medical student deeply engaged in global health since his undergraduate years at Berkeley ("Sujal Parikh," 2023). In 2009, Sujal received the Emerging Leader Award from Physicians for Human Rights; the next year he was appointed to their Student Advisory Board. He energized the Michigan global health community and we individually met on several occasions. On one of those occasions, he challenged me to become more personally active in support of social justice. It was the first time a student ever challenged me in the global health arena, and it was a truly inspiring and energizing moment for me. Sujal is the paradigm of the generation of students I envisioned in Chapter 11 when I suggested that students could be part of the leadership team of global health initiatives in the twenty-first century. His publications, for example, spanned new technologies, ethics and professionalism, and access to scholarly research (Parikh, 2010).

For many years I had been teaching an annual 120-person undergraduate course in women's reproductive health, and many students had gone on to medical school, schools of public health, nursing school, and midwifery school. Many of those who had gone to medical school pursued careers in women's health, and some even in global women's health. I spoke with them around once a year about advocacy and activism, especially in the context of abortion rights; sexual assault in the context of war, refugee status and interpersonal violence; and birthing choices. But Sujal was talking about more. He was talking about fully engaged advocacy. He was talking about an immersive activism that, despite all my years of active engagement in multiple successful programs in Ghana, I had failed to demonstrate. I had not taken advantage of the accomplishments of the Ghana program to push for broader attention to human rights and social justice; I had failed to do what my mentor and friend Doctor Allan Rosenfield had done with his 1985 article "Where is the M in MCH?" and sound a loud clarion call for women's sexual rights and reproductive justice. Although it has taken me a while to get it done, that was another reason for me to write this book. To tell the story that Mark Schlissel had wanted to hear. To leverage my work and what I think is a good story to encourage, inspire, and suggest approaches to new initiatives for new student activists, for a new generation of student advocates to pursue social justice, like Sujal Parikh. Sujal went on to receive a coveted Fogarty Fellowship to pursue his global health work in Kenya as a senior medical student and was tragically killed in a motorcycle accident there. An annual student-led symposium was created and named in his honor.

What should any student at any age and at any level who wants to pursue engaged global work do? They should first understand that they need to undertake developmentally appropriate experiences. Students who are freshman undergraduates are different than college seniors; first year medical students are different than fourth year students. Classwork, experiential learning, teaching experiences (e.g., Teach for America), research experience (e.g., Yaera Spraggins and Emma Lawrence), are all important to develop learners to become accomplished truly effective global leaders. It is not about medical tourism, medical voyeurism, or missionary work. This is about individual and, importantly, institutional behaviors and experiences that provide each learner with measurable, appropriate milestones and competencies.

> When I reflect on my own journey, which has focused on system strengthening in low-resource settings, I was propelled by experiences I had rotating as a student in the 1980s in India and Nepal. If I hadn't had those, I suspect that I wouldn't be spending the time working on global health that I do now. The point, though, that aligns with the premise is that the value in my experience as a student was not in providing care and assistance to those countries where I was rotating. Rather, it was preparing me and I was, in fact, getting much more out of it than I was giving. And the way forward is to expose other learners in a way that maximizes benefit [to host countries] and minimizes the harms that can result if these experiences aren't carefully thought through.
>
> Joseph C. Kolars, MD, senior associate dean for
> education and global Initiatives at UM Medical School,
> Josiah Macy, Jr., Professor of Health Professions
> Education (Michigan Medicine, 2016)

What should students do? They should demand that universities offer these opportunities in a pedagogically serious and ethically constructed way. This means universities need to provide established, ethically driven programs. This may often mean they need to use university funds or raise the university funds through philanthropy to support important programmatic global work and experiences. Students need to be advocates for this. Student voices are increasingly heard and listened to; the very students engaged in global programs can be the change advocates and activists not only globally but also by holding their own institutions to the ethical and behavioral standards that have been described and illustrated repeatedly in this book.

> Our approach to partnering with low- and middle- income countries and lower-resource settings than the United States is to build a platform that is jointly constructive to our partners. Partners are meaningful collaborators. They help create and drive the agenda. We collaborate within the creative platform of mutual benefits. We developed one for over 30 years in Ghana, where the premium is on capacity building, and we've had remarkable success.
>
> Brent Williams, MD, associate professor of
> internal medicine, director of the UM Medical
> School Global Health and Disparities Path of
> Excellence (Michigan Medicine, 2016)

Students need to demand that global health opportunities are available to students equitably on both sides of the partnership regardless of financial, racial, and other disparities. Throughout this book I have given non-US examples of global engagement, but there are real opportunities for students to do truly global work in areas of economic, racial, and ethnic disparity in the United States. Much of what we have thought about in the past as global has involved geographically extensive transnational or transcontinental travel, but many domestic experiences of an authentically "other" nature would qualify as equally "global" and transformative. Many students come to me and say they cannot afford to go abroad but are seeking a global experience. For some students I suggest they explore opportunities with underserved and underresourced populations in Michigan cities like Detroit or Muskegon, where there are huge disparities in income and access to health care. For others, I suggest they experience rural Michigan or the vast Upper Peninsula, both areas facing economic hardship, major issues with access to health care, and an epidemic of deadly substance use disorder. But even these domestic "global" experiences must be approached carefully by students who are developmentally and educationally prepared for them; and, in my opinion, they are best offered by universities following the same Charter principles that were highlighted in Chapter 8 and reinforced by illustrations throughout the narratives of this book. Students should demand these living learning opportunities as part of a liberal arts or a preprofessional education.

Health as a human right is a disruptive and transformative idea. Social justice is a disruptive and transformative idea. When we think about academic global health within the short-term context of the UN Sustainable Development Goals of 2015 to 2030 (see Chapter 11), and in the longer-term framework of human rights and social justice, we must do so strategically, opportunistically, and ethically. That is the message, the moral, and the challenge of the story of the Carnegie Ghana Postgraduate Training Programme in Obstetrics and Gynaecology.

Appendix 1

Charter

Anderson F et al. Creating a charter of collaboration for international university partnerships: the Elmina Declaration for Human Resources for Health. Academic Medicine: Journal of the Association of American Medical Colleges 89(8): 1125–32, 2014.

The Elmina Declaration on Partnerships to Address Human Resources for Health From the Ghana-Michigan Collaborative Health Alliance Reshaping Training, Education, and Research, 2009

Preamble: This document is a Charter for Collaboration which describes the partnership between groups working in Michigan, USA and Ghana to improve human resources for health funded by the Bill and Melinda Gates Foundation

The Elmina Declaration on Partnerships to Address Human Resources for Health From the Ghana-Michigan Collaborative Health Alliance Reshaping Training, Education & Research (CHARTER) Program

Initiated Elmina, Ghana 2–6 February, 2009

Adopted Ann Arbor, MI 8–13 November, 2009

We, the Ghana-Michigan CHARTER collaborators made up of partners from the Ghana Ministry of Health (MOH), the Kwame Nkrumah University of Science and Technology (KNUST), the University of Ghana (UG) (the three aforementioned heretofore referred to as Ghana) and the University of Michigan (UM),

I. Recognize that

1. Human Resources for Health (HRH) includes doctors, nurses, dentists, pharmacists, social workers, and other health professionals, both formal and informal, that are trained across the country by the Ministry of Health, the Ministry of Education, and the private sector.
   1. The burden of disease in Ghana requires a prioritization of HRH initiatives
   2. The Ghana-Michigan CHARTER project is a part of a larger HRH initiative in Ghana
   3. There are inadequate numbers and an asymmetric distribution of human resources in Ghana due to low numbers trained, urban concentration, and low retention of workers
   4. There is potential for growth in human resources for health in Ghana as evidenced by the high percentage of qualified applicants not gaining acceptance into training institutions
   5. Technological infrastructure is inadequate to support human resources for health and health service delivery, especially in the rural areas
   6. Traditional medicine is an important source of primary care for Ghanaians
2. Opportunities abound in our global community for HRH development
   1. Technological advances have promise to improve access to information for health workers and health students in all parts of Ghana, especially in rural areas, to improve education, service delivery, and advance research
   2. The private sector has many resources that could be harnessed to improve HRH
   3. Millennium Development Goals serve as a guide for research for health and health-related issues
   4. Prior experiences are a rich source of knowledge to explore, learn from, and share

5. Our partnerships are dynamic and may change over time; gaining knowledge and moving frontiers

6. We have an active commitment on the part of all partners to work together

3. Partnership and Collaboration are crucial for the Universities' and Ministry's shared mission and common interest in improving health outcomes

   1. The improvement of HRH requires "a new partnership" which calls for continuous planning, participation, assessment, and improvement

   2. Previous partnerships between Ghana and the University of Michigan have been successful, have led to other partnerships, and will continue to have impact at the community level

   3. Universities and the MOH have strategic plans and priorities that need to be considered, respected, and promoted

   4. The MOH has made a conscious effort with development partners to reduce verticalization. This project represents one of many development partnerships, and Ghana will work with their partners in a coordinated manner to optimize development and health

   5. Health teams include other allied health and health related professionals

4. Barriers exist in the development of partnerships to improve HRH

   1. Past partnerships have too often not been fair, balanced, equitable, or sustainable and have led to power imbalances between the Southern institutions and those in the North

   2. Barriers to growth of human resources exist, including: training opportunities, availability of housing, local teachers, infrastructure, other social structures

   3. The resources for electronic communication are not equal among all partners

4. There are infrastructure barriers: faculty promotion, communication, reporting systems, organizational structures, and managerial systems. Competition and financial structures, including compensation and release time, impact how work is accomplished. Structures of coordination are lacking in many partners

5. Individuals and institutions have histories and culture that bind them together but may keep them from breaking free to new ideas

6. Cultural heterogeneity exists between partners, and when there are failures, it can sometimes be attributed to these differences not being taken into account

7. The historical, social, and political context informs how service delivery and research are conducted

8. Research data are limited and exchange of information between academia and the MOH is inconsistent

9. There is potential for conflict between and within partners

10. Although we share a common language, operational definitions differ. Our common language creates the illusion of communication while misunderstandings still occur

11. Leadership structures can be challenging

II. Conscious of the need to

1. Share experiences in medical education, research, innovative technology, and leadership among all partners

2. Develop and share technological and other educational resources efficiently and effectively

3. Develop resources to optimize and fully utilize education, training, and deployment of HRH

4. Improve the infrastructure for electronic communication, skills training, and clinical care

5. Expand the scope of research and translate research results into policy and educational initiatives

6. Recognize, identify, and involve appropriate HRH workers in the process
7. Expand and decentralize education and training into peripheral health facilities, district, public, and private
8. Develop a national government research infrastructure to fund national health research
9. Articulate principles that guide partnerships to lead to sustainable, mutually beneficial collaboration, namely:

TRUST MUTUAL RESPECT COMMUNICATION
ACCOUNTABILITY TRANSPARENCY
LEADERSHIP
SUSTAINABILITY

III. Institutional Commitments

In pursuit of our determination to help improve the health of all Ghanaians through our objectives of enhancing education and training, strengthening data for decision making, and increasing capacity for research

We commit to:

1. Work together to create new knowledge and disseminate our findings through peer-reviewed literature and other means and use the results of our research to inform policy and decision making
2. Providing resources, both human and monetary, for understanding and learning from the partnerships through the development of the Charter for Collaboration document
3. Pursue funding for implementation of the findings from our projects with the overall goal of improving the health of all Ghanaians

4. Pursue and promote the increased use of information and communication technology and develop a communication plan to ensure frequent and open communication for all parties between and within institutions to address the needs of the partnership and objectives, including regular meetings, an accessible website, electronic communication, reports and others

5. Improve and facilitate communication: government to government, government to the academy (universities), academy to academy, and with the private sector, social leaders (churches, NGOs) and the community to maintain a balance in these partner relationships

6. Identify and protect the interests and needs of all partners and work towards meeting these needs

7. Create opportunities for personnel from the universities and Ministry of Health for career development

8. Develop authorship guidelines to promote fair and equitable recognition of individual and group contributions

9. Apply lessons learned from previous collaborations to inform current and future partnerships

10. Be sensitive to issues of gender, ethnicity, religion, and geographic origin

11. Organize and participate in a process to engage all partners currently working in the area of HRH to reduce verticalization and promote lateralization

12. Focus on early recognition of potential sources of conflict and develop a plan for identifying, recognizing, and managing conflicts

13. Evaluate the process on a regular basis and make adjustments accordingly

14. Establish metrics of successful collaborations by which to give feedback to our project

15. Document case examples of collaborative strains and successes

Appendix 2

The Bight of Benin and Beyond by J. B. Lawson

J.B. Lawson
(with a prologue by T.R.B. Johnson)

Ponteland, Newcastle upon Tyne, NE20 9RQ (UK)
(Received August 1st, 1990)
(Revised and accepted September 15th, 1990)

Prologue

The Nicholson J. Eastman Professorship was established by former students, residents and friends to honor Dr. Eastman, one of America's most influential and important obstetricians who served for more than 20 years as Obstetrician-in-Chief of the Johns Hopkins Hospital. Dr. Eastman spent two extended periods at the Beijing Union Medical College before succeeding Dr. J. Whitridge Williams in this position. In addition to his clinical duties and extensive teaching, Eastman edited the 10th, 11th, and 12th editions of Williams' Obstetrics and was editor for almost 20 years of Obstetric and Gynecologic Survey. It is appropriate for John Lawson to be the 1990 Eastman Professor. Professor Lawson, during his distinguished career, has been Professor of Obstetrics and Gynecology at the University of Ibadan, Nigeria from 1953—1969 and from 1981 to 1989, was Director of Postgraduate Studies at the Royal College of Obstetricians and Gynecologists. Obstetrics and Gynecology in the Tropics and Developing Countries remains the standard text in the field and is currently in revision with Dr. Kelsey Harrison as coauthor. The International Journal is pleased to publish this important and inspirational lecture which highlights two obstetrician/ gynecologists who continue to have international influence.

T.R.B. Johnson

I feel very honored to have been invited to give this lecture in memory of Professor Nicholson J. Eastman. He brought modern obstetrics to us through his splendid editions of Williams' Obstetrics (my bible in my early years) and when I met him in London in the 1960s, the enthusiastic encouragement he gave me was no doubt because I was following the same arduous road in Nigeria that he had traversed in China a generation earlier, endeavoring to develop modern obstetrics in a strange environment.

I thought obstetrics in the context of the wider world would be a subject of which Eastman would have approved and chose as title "The Bight of Benin and Beyond." The Bight of Benin is a prominent feature of the coastline of West Africa where Nigeria meets the Atlantic. There, after an all-too-short postgraduate training in England, I went in 1953 to help develop the first University in West Africa at Ibadan. From very small beginnings, a department of obstetrics and gynecology was built up. Later, a great hospital was built, students were taught, postgraduates trained and locally relevant research

0020-7292/90/$03.50
© 1990 International Federation of Gynecology and Obstetrics
Published and Printed in Ireland

Special Article

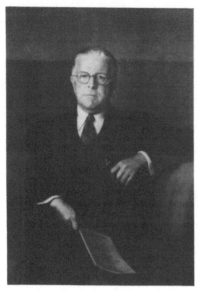

Nicholson J. Eastman

initiated during my next 17 years. From this experience, my interests widened to the maternal health problems of the Third World in general.

We delivered 5500 patients in the two years 1953—1954, nearly 20% of whom had received no antenatal care and who only came to the hospital because of serious complications. The casualties were horrific: 76 maternal deaths and 750 babies lost. Even among those who had received antenatal care of a sort, the maternal mortality was 5/1000. Why did they die?

The first answer is the most important one: almost all the maternal deaths could have been prevented by widely deployed maternity services of good quality in the community and by good communications.

The second lesson is that the deaths were not due to exotic tropical diseases. For the great killers are universal — difficult labor, sepsis, hemorrhage, eclampsia. In addition, severe anemia was an important contributor in Ibadan.

The third lesson is that the absence of stored blood for transfusion crippled us when trying to salvage obstetric emergencies. It continued to do so until we organized a safe blood bank later — the first in West Africa.

The fourth lesson is that our treatment methods, although no doubt appropriate for our previous lives in London, needed much modification in the light of our new experience. We had to learn a new trade. Let me give you some examples of what we learned about familiar obstetric conditions with unfamiliar features in tropical Africa.

Pre-eclampsia and eclampsia

Pre-eclampsia is considerably less common during pregnancy in tropical Africa than in the United Kingdom, but it develops more readily during labor. Pre-eclampsia appears to progress more rapidly to eclampsia, particularly in labor, in contrast to the more chronic course which is common in Europe. Fits occur at deceptively low blood pressure levels, 20% at a blood pressure of 140/90 or below and only one-third of eclamptics reach 160/100. Eclamptic fits are therefore much more difficult to prevent but the prognosis for the fetus is surprisingly good, no doubt because there is little time for placental damage to develop.

Cephalopelvic disproportion

In developing countries in the tropics, malnutrition and uncontrolled infections in childhood and adolescence commonly cause delayed development and stunting of growth of future mothers. Many women therefore fail to achieve their genetically determined stature. Contracted pelvis is accordingly much more common than in the United Kingdom. A serious additional factor in Muslim Northern Nigeria is too early a start to childbearing. Marriage soon after the menarche, followed by pregnancy before the young mother's pelvis is fully grown, increases the incidence of cephalopelvic disproportion.

Obstructed labor

I define obstruction to mean a labor in which progress is arrested by mechanical factors and delivery is impossible without operative assistance. Although modern obstetric care and increasing rarity of severely contracted pelvis have led to the virtual disappearance of obstructed labor from your obstetric scene, obstructed labor and its sequelae are the most important causes of maternal mortality in tropical Africa. Unhappily, the extension of modern obstetric care there affects those with the worst prognosis last.

Exhausted, dehydrated and infected women admitted in obstructed labor pose most difficult obstetric problems. With the uterus in tonic contraction, the fetus is usually already dead; the lower segment is dangerously stretched and spontaneous rupture may be imminent if it has not already occurred. When the uterus ruptures, maternal death can only be prevented by massive transfusion and immediate laparotomy.

Even when the unfortunate woman survives an obstructed labor, serious complications may follow. In particular, pressure necrosis may result in sloughing of the soft tissues impacted between the presenting part and the pelvic wall, causing vesico-vaginal and rectovaginal fistulas and the consequent miseries of incontinence. For the gynecologist practicing in tropical Africa, these conditions, which were not uncommon in the United Kingdom and the United States 100 years ago, still present the greatest surgical challenge.

Anemia

Anemia is the most important complication in pregnancy in tropical Africa, not only because of its greatly increased incidence, but also because of the severity with which it presents. It was eventually established that chronic hemolysis due to *P. falciparum* malaria infection was the root cause (during pregnancy the immunity acquired in childhood by recurrent infections declines). We demonstrated conclusively in a carefully controlled study, the efficacy of preventing anemia in pregnancy with antimalarials.

In some cases, the patients may die either undelivered or in the first two weeks of the puerperium. The main cause of death is congestive heart failure due to myocardial oxygen lack when the anemia is profound (hemoglobin level of 4 or below).

Apart from the direct effects of anemia, indirectly it influences maternal prognosis by making even small blood losses at delivery highly dangerous and by diminishing resistance to infection during the puerperium.

It also adversely affects the fetal prognosis. Midtrimester abortions and premature labors are common: intrauterine growth is impaired, resulting in lower birthweights at term. Severe maternal hypoxia may cause intrauterine death before the onset of labor or stillbirth or early neonatal death from intrapartum asphyxia.

In those early years, my colleagues and I learned what to teach our students and postgraduates about local clinical problems in the same way, I am sure, as Eastman did. At the same time, we learned about the local social and cultural influences on the phenomena of reproduction, many of which are highly adverse. It is clear to me that the disappointing progress in curbing the high maternal and infant casualty rates in the Third World is due to the persistence of these adverse factors.

What can be done to mitigate them? In all developing countries, lack of confidence in modern medical care, even when it is available, keeps patients away from doctors until their diseases are very advanced. This is especially true in obstetrics as the mysteries of birth resist new ideas to the last. The traditional conduct of labor by unskilled attendants adds to this by causing delay in the presence of dystocia or hemorrhage; isolation

Special Article

and poor communications worsen this delay.

However, as Kelsey Harrison has shown, raising the status of women by providing primary education results in increased confidence in and utilization of maternity services. So our problem is to make these services available in an acceptable form where they are needed — no easy task in the predominantly rural societies of the Third World.

How? Should more specialist obstetricians be provided? Having been Director of Postgraduate Studies at the Royal College of Obstetricians for six years, my answer in the negative may surprise you. I am very disappointed by the small contribution to improving maternal health in developing countries made by the large number of their nationals trained in Europe and America. Exclusive concentration on solving the clinical problems of individual patients does not fit the Third World trainee for leadership in maternity care on the bedrock of preventive medicine after his return home.

So, is there any need for more doctors in Third World countries at all? Yes, if they are better trained and better selected there than now. This must be based on understanding of and sympathy with the poor and the unemancipated, not just the affluent urban middle class.

Concentration on the old fashioned educational virtues is needed: careful history taking, methodical clinical technique, accurate records — all learned from good role models. Laboratory investigations come last in this litany because of their limited availability and limited reliability in developing countries. Do not misunderstand me. Of course I do not underrate the advantages of practicing with the help of the fetal monitor, the pH meter and the ultrasonograph, but I must insist that good medicine can be practiced without high technology if need be. (In the early days in Ibadan, our high-tech was limited to the microscope.)

But maternal morbidity and mortality in the Third World will not be conquered by

good basic doctors without further training. The district centers to which potential difficulties and complicated cases are referred for treatment from the periphery (Centers of First Referral in WHO terms), must be manned by general duty doctors who have been trained on the job to provide WHO's Essential Obstetric Functions. How to remove a placenta, evacuate an abortion, delivery by ventouse or craniotomy, or by cesarean section under local anesthesia are essential skills to be learned. Extending antenatal care, reducing high-risk factors like high parity or pregnancies when too young are all very well. They help, but they do not save individual lives: that needs competent emergency treatment by the trained medical officer in the district center.

So far, we have only discussed doctors, but the luxury of a doctor to personally attend every woman in pregnancy and labor as in the United States, is not an attainable target. For this, we need well trained midwives, educated, resourceful women who can take personal responsibility for the normal pregnancy and delivery and identify the signs of trouble for timely referral to a doctor with appropriate skills.

Nicholson Eastman knew all about this when the need for basic maternity services in what were then called "underdeveloped" countries was surveyed by the Expert Committee on Maternity Care of the World Health Organization which first met in Geneva in 1951 under his chairmanship. Four years later he chaired the WHO Expert Committee on Midwifery Training and I quote from his 1955 report:

The lack of medical and trained midwifery personnel in large areas of the world was discussed by the committee. The traditional birth attendant, untrained and the auxiliary midwife, slightly trained, are being used to help make up this deficiency. A program must be set up that will result in evolution from the use of the TBA and the auxiliary attendant to the fully qualified midwife. The increase in personnel will not provide better protection of the women of childbearing age, unless the training of the midwife is broadened to include sufficient knowledge and understanding to give prenatal, perinatal and postnatal care. This necessitates some knowledge of public health and certain nursing skills.

In sketching in categories of health workers to be involved in the provision of maternity care in developing countries where at present there is so little, I do not imply that the categories are separate. All are trying to do the same thing — provide safe motherhood for the community — so it is essential they work as a team. In each district, the midwives (and for the time being, well supervised TBAs) must be directed and coordinated from the district center. This will be the obstetric unit of the district hospital or the maternity center to which the potentially abnormal and the complicated cases will be referred. The leadership of the team will be provided by the well trained medical officer to be based there, who will give inspiration and teaching to those working in the area served.

Now you may think I am moving from the clinical concerns of obstetricians to social and organizational matters which are not our business. But indeed they are and it is perhaps in how to provide modern maternity care universally that our teaching is most deficient. Our practice is still targeted to individual mothers most readily available and receptive — the educated, the relatively affluent, those living in towns — people like us. Our target should be the less fortunate mothers who receive less than their due — and die as a result — all over the world. I am sure that Nicholson J. Eastman would have approved of that.

Address for reprints:

T.R.B. Johnson
Eastman Professor Office
Houck 228, Johns Hopkins Hospital
600 North Wolfe Street
Baltimore, MD 21205, USA

Appendix 3

TRAVEL TIPS FOR VISITORS TO GHANA!

Last Updated January, 2023

DOCUMENTS NEEDED FOR ENTRY:
1. **Current passport** with blank pages. Application process takes about 3 weeks. You can get the application at the U.S. Post Office. Photos can be done at many copy shops or most drugstore chains.
2. **Visa for Ghana**
   a. Generally, apply for a **"tourist" visa (B1/B2)**, "single entry" (can only enter Ghana once). If you anticipate wanting to travel to surrounding countries and return to Ghana, or anticipate making additional trips to Ghana in the next 5 years, select the "multiple entry" option.
   b. See website for details - options:
      i. https://www.ghanaembassydc.org/visas
      ii. https://ecimsglobal.com/mission.aspx
   c. These get mailed to the Ghanaian embassy in Washington DC or New York and they stamp your visa in your passport and return to you. Takes about 1-3 weeks.
   d. Follow directions carefully - can be confusing and changes often
3. **Certificate of immunization against yellow fever** (generally this is provided by the Travel Clinic)

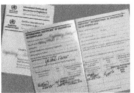

4. **COVID-specific info:** *(current as of June 2022, check updated guidelines with airline and embassy:*
   https://gh.usembassy.gov/ghana-covid-19-information/#:~:text=Individuals%20arriving%20in%20Ghana%20by,72%20hours%20prior%20to%20departure.)

   a. Need COVID vaccination card to enter
   b. IF vaccinated, do not need covid testing to arrive

HEALTH
- Make an appointment as early as possible with a travel clinic.
- Required vaccines: Yellow fever; COVID-19
   o You need proof of updated yellow fever vaccination with a "yellow fever card" to enter the country!

- Recommended vaccinations: up to date on HepA, Hepatitis B, tetanus booster, polio booster, typhoid, meningitis.
- Check the CDC travel website for current health recommendations or any outbreaks which you should be aware of
- Take with you to Ghana:
    - Preventive malaria medication (malarone and doxycyline are typical favorites)
    - Azithromycin (for travelers diarrhea; only take if symptomatic with >3 loose stools in 8 hours)
    - Acetaminophen and/or ibuprofen
    - Thermometer
    - Antibiotic ointment (easy skin infections in tropical weather)
    - Band-aids
    - Personal medications you may be on (in original rx bottles)
    - Imodium (treatment for diarrhea)
    - Pepto bismol (taking it daily cuts risk of travelers diarrhea in half)
    - Mosquito repellent with 30-50% DEET.
    - Antihistamines (for severe mosquito bites)
    - Sunscreen / sunglasses
- You can find/buy almost anything you need in Ghana. There are lots of pharmacies around the hospital areas, which sell all range of medications. There are some cheap knockoff medications, so ask the pharmacist for the best quality. **Tampons**, contact lens solutions, and sunscreen are harder to find, but shoprite (in Accra and Kumasi) is a good bet to find a wide range of Western items
- Malaria nets/tents to sleep under are not necessary in mid/upper range hostels/hostels. May be worth bringing if you are planning to "rough it" and spend time outside the cities in places without screened windows.

TIME
Ghana is 4-5 hours ahead of US Eastern time zone. (Ghana does not observe daylight savings)

MONEY:
- The local currency is the Cedi - the exchange rates are constanting changing so check before you travel
- You will need cash for daily purchases (and paying for non-high range hotels and restaurants); two best approaches:
    - Bring USD cash and exchange for cedis at a bank in Ghana
        - Larger bill ($100s) and newer bills (dates <10 years old) will get better exchange rates
    - Use your debit card at ATMs in Ghana to withdraw cedis
        - Check with your bank about international transaction fees
        - There are ATMs at every corner in major cities, including two large collections of ATMs just outside Korle Bu and KATH hospitals

- Visa is the best option. Just look for the visa symbol on ATM (American Express is not often accepted; Mastercard is sometimes accepted)
- Credit card fraud is a risk in Ghana and you should use your credit card sparingly (only if you can keep tabs on your credit card statements/usage; using at major hotels and shopping malls is usually ok).
- Contact your credit/debit card(s) company and/or bank ahead of time so they don't place holds on your cards when they are used in Ghana.
- Traveler's checks are not widely accepted and not recommended for Ghana.
- A reasonable approach is to take with you: credit card x1, debit card x1 (bring a second if you have one for a backup) and $200 in USD. If you don't have a visa debit card or there will be high fees, then bring enough USD cash to exchange into cedis to cover your hotel and daily needs.

GETTING TO GHANA:
- There are several major airlines that fly to Accra, Ghana (Kotoko airport), including Delta.
- You are allowed 2 checked bags to fly international. Take advantage of this – pack lightly, take 2 large bags (filled only half-way each, perhaps) so as to have room to bring home all the souvenirs you will pick up.

IN-COUNTRY TRANSPORTATION:
- Safety
  - Walking is generally safe but be cautious in rural areas, when alone, and certainly after dark, even though Ghana is a relatively safe country.
  - Driving is one of the most risky activities you will face in Ghana. Avoid traveling cross-country at nighttime if possible, especially if traveling alone.
  - Avoid riding on motor scooters and motorcycles as these are also very high risk for accidents
- Flights
  - There are domestic flights, currently between Accra, Kumasi, Tamale, and Takoradi. A more expensive but must quicker way to transit between major cities.
  - There are multiple domestic carriers, including Africa World Air and Passion Air.
  - Schedules are posted online and tickets can be reserved online. Currently, flights need to be paid for in cash at the airport, but this may change in the near future.
  - In Accra, there are separate international and domestic terminals, located a short walk from one another
- Uber and Bolt
  - As of ~2020, Uber and Bolt have replaced taxis as the easiest and most common for local travel in major cities.
  - Use the app the same way as you would in the USA. You need a smartphone with a connection to the internet to use. The cars are typically comfortable, a bit cheaper than taxis, and eliminate the stress of bargaining

- o   You can pay by credit card or by cash (drivers will prefer cash and may reject rides paid with card).
- Taxi
    - o   Taxis have no meters in them. Price is decided upon before you get in, so don't accept the ride until you have negotiated. Be prepared to negotiate, as drivers often hike the going rate by 2-3 times if they know you are a visitor. Before catching a taxi, ask a local how much they anticipate a ride should cost, so you are prepared to bargain.
    - o   Taxis may or may not have seatbelts
    - o   Hotels can often help arrange a driver for you but is likely to be about 3x whatever price you would arrange with a taxi (though often in a car which is nicer and safer).
    - o   Faculty may find themselves escorted by hospital drivers who will be sent to pick them up and dispatched to take them back to the hotel in the evening.
- Tro-tros
    - o   Seen everywhere in Ghana, these are over-packed mini-busses that run fixed routes within and between cities. Passengers can hop off and on anywhere along the root, with inexpensive fares. The "mate" will call out the destination.
    - o   Typically crowded and not comfortable. The least expensive travel option, but difficult to navigate if you don't know the routes well.
- Buses
    - o   There are several reliable and very comfortable bus services (OA, STC, VIP) that run at scheduled times between major cities. These coach buses have space for luggage below (for a small fee) and you can carry a small bag on with you. They have air con and reclining seats. This is a longer but cheaper alternative to air travel.
    - o   Each major city has stations where you can purchase bus tickets. It is recommended to purchase tickets several days ahead of planned travel since they can fill up.

MEDICAL INSURANCE

- For visitors from University of Michigan, UMHS recommends a couple of options for emergency medical evacuation insurance. Options include Medex SafeTrip and Travel Health International through the UMMS Office of Student Programs.
- Travel insurance is required by UM for any student traveling abroad for elective.

PHONE

- It is essential to have a cell phone in Ghana, even if you don't use or need one in the United States. This is the primary form of communication, even within the hospital as there is rarely any other type of phone available for use and no pagers.

- Some cell phones have international options, so may be worth checking with your plan; however, it can be expensive
- It is recommended to buy a local SIM card so you can communicate easily/cheaply with others in Ghana using the local network. Local networks include MTN, Vodofone, etc. SIM cards, as well as additional credit to add to your card when you run out, are available everywhere. In the rare exception of a very long stay where you pay for a plan, the vast majority of travelers (and Ghanaians) use a pay as you go approach where you add phone credit as needed for calls, texts, and data for internet use. You can either purchase a phone in Ghana (everything from iphones or basic non-smart phones are available) or use your personal phone in Ghana (as long as it's "unlocked" and you can remove the sim card)
- Phones and SIM cards are sold at the airport upon arrival, and throughout all major cities. *You need your passport to buy a Ghanaian sim card.*

INTERNET / COMPUTERS

- Every year, internet becomes faster and more accessible. Options change/improve every year so ask your local contacts for the best new options!
- If you are using a smart phone with a local carrier, you can purchase credit to use as data and have reasonably fast internet on your phone. This is nice for using Uber, google maps, etc.
- For your laptop, you can buy a wireless USB stick (portable modem) from a local carrier which allows you to connect to the internet. It emits a wireless signal and can be shared among anyone close by. They generally come preloaded with a reasonable amount of starting data.
- There are internet cafes throughout major cities. The MTN and Vodofone cafes have air con and are very fast. There is wifi at update hotels. For non-guests, you can pay to use the wifi (and the pool).
- Internet access at the hospitals is fairly limited. Korle Bu and KATH both have libraries, which have air con and are a nice place to work. Wifi is sometimes working :).
- Most visitors bring their personal laptop
- Viruses are RAMPANT. Be very careful of sharing files, using stick drives, etc. Invest in anti-virus software and make sure it's up to date.

PACKING:

HOSPITAL/CLINICAL WORK

- Nametag / ID
- Notebook / pens
- Stethoscope, penlight, reflex hammer, etc (any other diagnostic tools frequently used in your specialty)
- Eye protection
- Surgical caps
- Personal masks for daily hospital use; consider bringing N95 masks

- Hand sanitizer
- Hospital/clinic attire:
    - White Coat
    - 2-3 pairs of Scrubs (students/residents bring their own scrubs to the hospital); needed for labor and delivery/OR/ED
    - Operating room shoes if you will be in the OR
        - Need a separate pair of shoes than the ones you were wearing to/around the hospital; often crocs or plastic clogs
    - Clothes for hospital rounding and clinics:
        - In general, dress as you would for your own clinic on a very hot day without air-conditioning. The hospitals tend to be mostly open-air, without air-conditioning, and hot and humid.
        - Men should plan to wear long dress pants, dress shoes or sandals (most Ghanaian men have closed-toed sandals or regular casual shoes), short-sleeved collared cotton shirts. Men should take a tie. For formal events, jackets are worn but you should be fine with a short-sleeved cotton shirt +/- tie for most work things.
        - Women should wear to/below-the-knee pants, capris or skirts/dresses. Cotton t-shirts or blouses and skirts/pants will be the most comfortable.

CLOTHING

- Bring a swimsuit as the major hotels have nice pools. If you are not staying in a hotel with a pool, you can often pay a day fee to swim
- A very light linen or cotton jacket since it can be cold in air-conditioned settings like hotels, meeting rooms, buses
- Casual clothing: Bring sandals with a sturdy sole for exploring the markets and town. It's hot, so loose breathable clothing is recommended! For woman, sundresses, skirts (to the knee), and shirts that show bare shoulders are fine. However, short skirts and short shorts are not appropriate outside of your hotel.
- For shoes wear daily walking sandals or closed-toe shoes; recommend closed toed shoes in the hospital. You will probably not be comfortable in high heels, strappy shoes, or wearing shoes which require socks.
- Some option for breathable long sleeves/long pants to wear in national parks where the mosquitoes are fierce.
- NOTE: if you have any open sores or cuts on your feet, cover them with bandaids or wear closed shoes.
- LAUNDRY: Clothing can be washed by the hotel (for a fee) or you can plan to hand-wash in the sink (powdered detergent is easy to find). You will be happiest with fabrics which dry quickly and don't need ironing.

OTHER ITEMS TO PACK:

- Bring a shoulder bag or tote/briefcase to carry papers, computer, Deet, Kleenex, water bottle, etc.

- Take plug/converter(s). You may need 2 different types of plug adaptors (one with 2 prongs and one with 3) but you can often find a multi-plus adaptor which works for many countries, including all the plug types for Ghana.
  - For Ghana there are two associated plug types, D and G. Plug type D is the plug which has three round pins in a triangular pattern and type G is the plug which has three rectangular pins in a triangular pattern

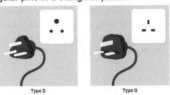

Type D   Type G

- You may or may not find a blow dryer at the hotels so may wish to pack one.
- Do take a travel alarm clock or be prepared to use the alarm on your cell phone. Most hotels surprisingly do NOT even have clocks.
- If you will be at a hostel, consider luggage locks and laptop locks.
- Students should bring their MCard for hospital ID and for student discounts
- Some students have suggested travel speakers, small fan, flip flops for shared showers, ear plugs, and flashlight.
- You should bring some Ziploc bags, alcohol swabs or wet wipes.
- If you are a coffee drinker, you should bring a French Press (or alternate form of coffee maker) and coffee beans. Ghana is not known for its coffee and a morning cup of Joe is important.

WATER
- Use bottled water for brushing teeth, taking meds, etc. No water from the tap, shower, sink. NO ICE.
- On EVERY street corner, people sell bottles of water and cheaper alternatives (bags of water called sashays). You can also buy a large case of bottles water from any grocery store to keep in your room.
- Do carry a bottle of water with you during the day and be careful about getting dehydrated.

FOOD
- As of ~2020, food delivery apps are now popular and easy (similar to grubhub) in Accra, and potentially soon coming to other cities. Main ones include "Jumia" and "Glovo"
- One mantra to follow is: *peel it, boil it, cook it, or forget it.*
- Ghanaian food tends to be meat heavy although it is possible to eat vegetarian, particularly at the hotels and larger restaurants. The diet is mostly meat, fish, starches, and fruit. Virtually all soups are made with meat base.
- Ghanaian food also tends to be spicy.

- Avoid cold food, salads (washed in tap water), fruits other than those you have washed yourself in bottled water, salads, and salad items.
- Street food has mixed recommendations from guide books in terms of safety. If you eat food from street vendors, most recommended sticking with things which met the other criteria (ie hot food, fruits you peel, boiled eggs, cooked food, etc).
- There are several large grocery stores in Accra and Kumasi, ranging from local stores to Shoprite (more expensive but has full Western options)
- Consider packing a stash of nuts, dried fruit, protein bars, peanut butter, crackers, etc in your suitcase – sometimes it's just enough to tide you over, sometimes it's just enough to settle your stomach, sometimes it's just a nice reminder of home.

PLACES TO STAY
- There are upmarket hotel options in Accra and other major cities. In Accra, there are multiple international chains. In Kumasi, upmarket hotels include the Golden Tulip (now called "Lancaster") and Golden Bean. These are generally well above the budget of visiting students and residents, however most have a day pass where you can pay to enjoy the pool/lunch/internet. These all accept major credit cards.
- Medical hostel options in Accra
  - **International Student Hostel** at the University of Ghana which is located within the Korle Bu grounds. Not as nice as the Kumasi counterpart and does not have the benefit of being full of other local students. An ok option if you are looking for something budget friendly. Has fans and running water. No air con. No restaurant, which is a downside.
- Medical hospital options in Kumasi
  - **Medical Student Hostel ("Getfund") at KATH** is right next to the hospital within the compound. This is where the majority of Ghanaian medical students also stay. Rooms are basic, with two single beds, fan, bathroom with modern toilet and running shower. No A/C or hot water. Adjacent to the hostel restaurant which serves tasty and inexpensive meals. This is a fun way to get to know local medical students, and is very convenient! Recommend for visiting medical students doing an elective.
- Mid-range recommendation near KATH (Kumasi):
  - **Kumasi Catering Rest House:** Walking distance from KATH. Air/con, mini-fridge in the room, hot water, breakfast included, restaurant on site with good food, friendly staff, wifi (usually working).
  - https://www.aplacetostay.co/ghana/kumasi/kumasi-catering-rest-house
- Mid-range recommendation near Korle Bu (Accra):
  - **Nurses and Midwives Hostel:** More like a hotel than a "hostel." Close to Korle Bu (longer walk or a very short taxi/uber ride; many taxis passing through the junction just down the street). Very nice staff. Big rooms with air con, fan, minifridge, TV, private bathroom with hot water. Breakfast is included; has a restaurant that does now serve other meals.

- Dean's Guesthouse: Very close to hospital. Air con, fan, minifridge, TV, private bathroom with hot water. Breakfast is included, and restaurant is open for other meals.

SAFETY

- Ghana is a relatively safe country. Most guidebooks recommend against traveling alone, particularly in isolated areas, which seems pretty common-sense. If you are Caucasian you may sometimes be identified (and called) "obruni" which means "white person"
- Carry Xerox copies of your passport on your person rather than your actual documents (which you should leave in your locked luggage and in your locked hotel room).
- Many guidebooks recommend against wearing any jewelry or expensive watches.
- For women, expect a fair amount of extra hassle…but also some protectiveness. Women in particular should be cautious about walking alone at night.
- It is very common in Ghana for people to try to help you in a rather pushy way…to be your guide, carry bags, help escort you thru customs. You do not need this, so just be polite, cheerful, and firm in rejecting these frequent and recurrent offers.

SHOPPING

- Ghanaian vendors expect to negotiate and will set very high prices in areas where tourists visit and particularly for white tourists who will stand out. Some people liked to negotiate by asking the seller to name a price first and then offering half. Be polite and willing to negotiate a little but also willing to walk away as people may give in to your price when they see you are going to walk away without buying.
- In some settings which were more store-like, prices are set ("fixed")
- In the actual street markets, prices tended to be quite negotiable.
- Centers to buy handicrafts and paintings
  - The Arts Center in Accra - hectic with lots of hassling and bargaining, but great selection
  - The Cultural Center in Kumasi - lovely and quiet with walled in gardens; can watch the artisans work
- You can purchase local fabric either at the market or stores and take it to a tailor/dressmaker to have custom dresses and shirts made.

TOURISM

- Bradt Travel Guide to Ghana is a great guidebook and worth purchasing: https://www.amazon.com/Ghana-6th-Bradt-Travel-Guide/dp/1841624780
- CAPE COAST:
  - Regular buses run from other major cities (or you can rent a van and driver if traveling with a group)
  - Elmina Beach Resort hotel (15km from Cape Coast) is recommended upmarket option and Oasis Beach resort is a good budget option (right on the beach and has a popular restaurant and nightclub)
  - Cape Coast Castle: one of the largest forts for slave trade in Africa

- Kakum National Park 45 minutes from Cape Coast where you can do a canopy walk on a type of rope ladder, up over the forest. It is recommended that if you go to Kakum, you ask your taxi driver to wait for you or there may be no one around to take you back.
- TAMALE area:
    - Mole (moh-lay) National Park (Ghana's largest wildlife sanctuary) which requires another several-hour trip via tro-tro or STC bus for 45 minutes drive. You can see elephants, antelope, crocodiles, monkeys. At the park there is a hotel (Mole Motel) with a pool and restaurant that overlooks a valley with two watering holes visited by the animals. You can go on inexpensive walking and jeep safaris. Plan on staying the night if you go to the park.
    - From Tamale, Paga is a 2-3 hour drive north. Paga is where there are crocodiles hanging out amongst the animals and people, and you can get your picture taken with a crocodile.
- ACCRA:
    - Kwame Nkrumah Memorial Park
    - Arts Center for shopping
    - Lighthouse of Jamestown
    - National Museum
    - La Beach/Labadi Beach Resort
    - Local soccer matches
    - Bojo Beach: lovely quiet beach just out of town, worth the drive to escape the hassle and trash on some of the public beaches. You take a few minute row boat ride to get to the beach.
- KUMASI
    - Cultural center - shopping and watching local artisans work. Ike's cafe serves good food overlooking a pond
    - Central Market - one of the largest markets in Africa
    - Green Ranch - horseback riding and lovely vegetarian food at Lake Bosomtwe (https://www.greenranchlakebosomtwe.com/en/)
    - Bonwere Kenta Weaving Village
    - Ntonso Village: Edinkra Symbols Cloth Making
    - Ahwia Village: Wood Carving
    - Butterfly Sanctuary

PERSONAL/HEALTH
- The sun is very bright so be prepared with sunscreen when you are outside.
- You should plan on spraying yourself with 30-50% DEET solution or cream. In the rainy season, there are mosquitoes everywhere (even in the hospital and clinic), so don't assume that just because you will be inside there won't be mosquitoes. Malaria apparently presents with symptoms about 7-14 days after a bite but it may be as late as 6 months later. Common signs include headache, fever, chills, abdominal pain, and a

bitter taste in the mouth but can have a huge range of symptoms including fatigue, cough, nausea, and diarrhea. African mosquitoes are very small and you don't mount a typical local immune response (red, itchy bump) like you do in the U.S., so you often do not know you have been bitten.

- Avoid exposure to fresh water rivers due to the risk of schistosomiasis.
- Be cautious when walking along the ocean or other areas littered with trash. Wear shoes.
- Take a small container of Purell with you for use since soap is often unavailable.
- Do carry tissue with you everywhere as it is generally not available in restrooms.
- Do anticipate that you will have some GI distress and diarrhea at some point during the trip, most likely due to E.coli. If symptoms are severe, you can start taking cipro; if not severe, they may pass on their own in a day or two. It apparently takes 3-4 months to gain immunity to local strains of E.coli so it is not likely to happen during a short trip. The most important action is to maintain your hydration.
- Virtually all common prescription medications (malaria meds, inhalers, antibiotics) can be purchased without a prescription at any local pharmacy.

CULTURAL TIPS
- Ghanaians place a premium on greeting each other and saying hello. You would do well to have a small greeting (good morning, good evening, or how are you) prior to asking questions or asking for help.
- The bathroom is typically called the —washroom. You may want to carry a small amount of tissue with you as it is not always available.
- Fine to shake hands when you meet people but use your right hand. If you are in a group, it is considered polite to go in a counter-clockwise order as you shake hands.
- OK to take photos but be discreet. Many people do not like having their picture taken so ask permission. For patient care, often it is OK with the patient as long as you if you ask their permission first and if you let them (or the supervising doctor/nurse) know that you will not take a picture of their face—just the physical finding you are trying to document on their body. That seems to make it more acceptable. Do not take pictures of government or military instillations as this is against national law.
- Scheduled time is less punctual than you might anticipate. Clinic starts around the scheduled start time. Drivers will typically come exactly when they say (or even an hour early!) but hospital events, meetings, and rounds seemed quite relaxed and flexible in terms of starting time.
- Negotiate for prices BEFORE using a service. Settle on the final price (and what might or might not be included in the price, if appropriate) before a taxi ride, before a cross-country trip, before someone packs up a souvenir to sell you.
- Tipping is less common in Ghana. You might tip a driver you use frequently at the end of the week. Tipping is usually 10% at best. More expected in hotels, not in other settings. Restaurants sometimes include an automatic 15% gratuity in the bill which should be listed for you.

- Ghanaians refer to their close friends and associates with terms like "sister", "brother", "father";- 99.99 % of the time the person referred to in this way is not blood related. Get used to it and feel honored when you are referred to as one's sibling.

REVIEW OF MEDICAL TRAINING IN GHANA

- In Ghana, students start medical school directly after high school and embark on a six-year curriculum that encompasses courses in the basic sciences, public health, and core-clerkship experiences.
- After graduating, students become physicians and complete two house officer years in which they rotate through 4 specialties (OB/Gyn, Pediatrics, Internal Medicine, and Surgery) and manage patients on the wards.
- After their 2 years as house officers, trainees apply to residency (generally 3 years) in the field of their choice. This system is seen in many British Commonwealth countries, including India, and contrasts with the American system in which students typically complete four years of undergraduate studies, followed by four years of medical school, after which they are directed to their specific field of choice once they become resident physicians.
- There are two post-graduate colleges independently involved in training in Ghana. One is WACP, the West African College of Physicians, and one is GCPS, the Ghana College of Physicians and Surgeons. To become members of the Ghana College of Physicians and Surgeons, doctors must complete their fellowship, take the membership exam, serve time in the districts, and then do 18-24 more months of training in a sub-specialty and then take a Fellowship Exam.

POSSIBLE RESOURCES IN PREPARATION FOR TRAVEL

- GlobalREACH web site at UM has many resources on-line specific to medical school training, education, and research:
  http://www.med.umich.edu/medschool/globalreach/index.html
- Global REACH Student Handbook for Global Engagement:
  http://www.globalhealth.umich.edu/pdf/CGH%20standards%20handbook.pdf

ACKNOWLEDGEMENTS

Thank you to the following people who developed and reviewed the original document: Natalie Clark(Medical School), Dipa Joshi (Medical School), Cheryl Moyer (GlobalREACH), Pamela Rockwell (Family Medicine), Carrie Ashton (GlobalREACH), Jillian Plonsker (LSA-neuroscience), Kathleen Sienko (Engineering), Katie Gold (family medicine).

Travel Tips for Visitors to the University of Michigan: How to Prepare and What to Expect

Emergencies

Call 911 if you need immediate help in a life-threatening situation.

The dispatcher will ask you what type of emergency you are calling about. Respond that you need the police, fire department, or ambulance. The dispatcher will ask more questions, so do not hang up the phone.

Quick tips

- If you will be using credit cards when you are here please notify your credit card company that you will be traveling. Otherwise they could consider your purchases to be fraudulent.
- Be sure to have your invitation letter and any visa paperwork with you throughout your travels here. Do not pack it in your checked luggage.
- Bring one or more electrical plug converters
- Bring an umbrella
- Medical students should wear a short white lab coat. Physicians wear long white labcoats
- Your flights will be long so stay hydrated and sleep whenever you can!

- Bring US dollars. The first days here you will need to buy food, a bus pass, and possibly a local SIM card for your phone. Converting currency at local banks will incur a small charge.
- Bring your passport with you on your first day in the hospital. You will need it in order to get an ID badge.
- You can get a SIM card for your phone online that has a US telephone number.

Weather

https://www.usclimatedata.com/climate/ann-arbor/michigan/united-states/usmi0028

Packing

This website teaches you to pack efficiently and effectively – www.onebag.com .

If you take medication, bring enough for the entire visit. Some medications may only be available by prescription in the USA or unavailable completely.

If you layer your clothing, you will be ready for temperatures both inside and out.

Dress code for women: Professional dress is most appropriate. Dress pants, blouses, jackets, skirts, dresses. Short sleeved shirts are fine but should cover shoulders and under-arms. Sandals are fine. Shoes should be comfortable for walking/standing all day.

Avoid: t-shirts, jeans, shorts, tank tops, sun dresses, mini-skirts, low cut shirts, athletic shoes, beach shoes (flip-flops).

Dress code for men: Professional dress is most appropriate. Sport coat/blazer, Button down shirt (with or without a tie), dress pants or khaki pants, leather shoes. Wear shoes that are comfortable for walking/standing all day.

Avoid: t-shirts, jeans, shorts, tank tops, athletic shoes, beach shoes (flip flops)

Plan to pack clothing for casual days and lounging.

Fragrance policy

While in medical campus buildings do not wear perfume/cologne or strongly fragranced hair or body products. These products can irritate people with sensitivity.

Keep clothes and body clean to avoid objectionable odors.

Avoid smelling of cigarette smoke.

Smoking

Smoking is prohibited on all University of Michigan property, indoors and out. You must leave campus (go to a public outdoor area) in order to smoke.

There is no smoking allowed in any government building, restaurant, bar, or business.

There is no smoking allowed in taxis or public transportation.

Always ask permission before smoking in someone's vehicle or home.

US Customs and Culture

www.edupass.org Click on Cultural Differences and Living in the USA.

Personal distance and physical contact

Shaking hands upon meeting is customary. A firm handshake (neither squeezing hard nor too lightly) is ideal. In a health care setting you may not find as much hand shaking in order to prevent the spreading of germs.

Americans like a bit more personal space than many other cultures. People typically stand an arms-length away from each other when conversing.

Eye contact is considered normal and NOT a sign of disrespect. It indicates openness, honesty, and interest.

Taxes

In the state of Michigan there is a sales tax of 6% on all goods except unprepared food (grocery store). Restaurants do charge tax.

Tipping

A tip (or gratuity) of 15 – 20% is expected for the server when you dine in a restaurant or driver when you take a taxi. Tipping is not expected by the cashier at a fast food restaurant or other shops where you order at a counter.

Writing dates

Dates are written Month/Day/Year (8/10/1992). To avoid any confusion, it might be best to write out the date (August 10, 1992).

Electronics

Electric outlets operate with a voltage of 110-120 volts, 60 cycles. If your equipment requires 220 volts, bring a transformer. A plug converter will be needed for most visitors. Purchase one or more before you travel.

Type B

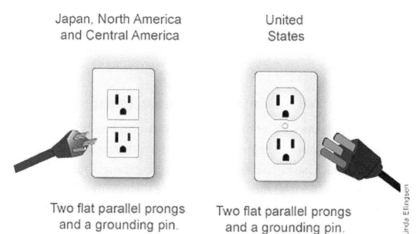

Japan, North America and Central America

United States

Two flat parallel prongs and a grounding pin.

Two flat parallel prongs and a grounding pin.

Linda Ellingsen

Prices are fixed

You cannot negotiate the price of items or services. The prices are fixed and either marked on the item with a sticker or shown by a sign on the store shelf. This includes taxis.

Punctuality

You should always be on time (or even a few minutes early) to a business meeting. Personal plans have more flexibility. If you are going to be late you should always call or send a message to the person waiting for you.

If someone is picking you up then you should be <u>ready to go</u> at that time.

Forms of address

In a professional setting address men as mister (Mr.), Doctor, or Professor. Women should be address as miss, missus, or miz (Ms.), Doctor, or Professor. Avoid using first names until invited to do so. But, do not use first names in the presence of patients.

In an informal setting Americans will typically introduce themselves by their first name, without titles. If you are introduced to someone by their first name then you may address him or her by their first name only.

When in doubt it is appropriate to ask someone their preference.

Personal information exchanges

It is ok to inquire about someone's family, children, hobbies, interests, etc. However, be careful not to ask questions that are too personal (Why aren't you married? Why don't you have children?). Politics and religion are often controversial topics. Conversely, Americans may share information with you that you consider highly personal.

Americans will often ask about your job during casual conversation or getting to know you. "What do you do?" means, what is your job/career?

Do not ask about someone's salary or how much they paid for something.

Getting and Using telephones

From a land line you must dial "1" before the area code and phone number.

Calling from one University telephone to another: Dial only the last 5 digits.

Calling from a University telephone to an outside number: check within the department to find out what number will access an "outside" line. In the Medical School it is "9". In the hospital it is "9-1".

Cell phones and SIM cards

AT&T store. 30 day plan for ~$60 (unlimited local talk and text plus data). International calling requires an additional calling card or addition to the plan. AT&T has an international package but not all countries are included. They have other less expensive packages depending on the phone and your needs. There is a store at 3217 Washtenaw Avenue by Barnes & Noble and a store in downtown at 407 E. Liberty Street. Blackberries cannot get a new local sim card.

T-mobile has similar packages. There's a store in the Briarwood Mall and one downtown at 200 E. Washington Street.

Best Buy. Buy a $20 phone and set up an account for 30 days at a time. They will set it up for you. There are more expensive phones with more features, internet, etc. There is a small version of Best Buy in the Briarwood Mall or the full sized store at 3100 Lohr Road.

Go Phone or similar from any CVS, Rite Aid, Walgreens, Kroger. This is the most expensive option per minute, but suitable for low usage users.

Campus Information Center

This site is a great starting point to find maps, transportation information, shopping, things to do, acronyms, museums, and other resources. https://campusinfo.umich.edu/

Transportation

Train
Amtrak www.amtrak.com

Bus routes and schedules
Ann Arbor Area Transportation Authority http://www.theride.org -
You can purchase a 30 day pass at Blake Transit Center for $58.
U-M bus routes and schedules https://ltp.umich.edu/transit/routes.php
    These are free.
Greyhound: www.greyhound.com
Megabus: www.megabus.com

To/From airport
Michigan Flyer: http://www.michiganflyer.com/
Takes you to Blake Transit Center
Ann Arbor Airport Shuttle: http://www.annarborairportshuttle.net/
Will take you to any address

Taxi
Across Town Cab
734-216-5932

Blue Cab
www.Bluecab.net
734-547-2222

Ann Arbor Taxi
http://www.annarbortaxi.com/
734-214-9999

Amazing Blue Taxi
734-846-0007

Ann Arbor Yellow Cab
734-663-3355

Metro Cab
734-997-6500

NightRide
This late-night, curb-to-curb taxi service operates within the City of Ann Arbor and east to downtown Ypsilanti between Clark Road/East Huron River Drive on the north and Ellsworth Road/Michigan Avenue on the south.

<u>When It Runs</u>

Monday – Friday: Midnight - 6am
Saturday: 11pm - 7:30am
Sunday 8pm - 7:30am
No trip requests are taken after 5:15am Monday – Friday (5am for trips outside of Ann Arbor) and 6:45am on Saturday/Sunday (6:30am outside of Ann Arbor). To reserve your ride, please continue to call 734-528-5432.

<u>How to Ride</u>

Advance reservations are strongly encouraged for trips that begin or end outside Ann Arbor.

Advance reservations can be made the day before your trip by calling 734-528-5432 or emailing nightride@theride.org.

Please provide the following trip information:

- Your name
- Your telephone number
- Earliest pick-up time
- Your pick-up location (Please specify, i.e. Garden Center Meijer)

- Location where you are going
- Number of passengers (including any non-paying children)
- If you are using a car seat or wheelchair
- If you want a call-back when the cab is arriving

Once you have made an advance reservation, **please call to confirm your trip at least 60 minutes before requested pickup time** (leave a message if this is before service begins).

You may stay indoors until the NightRide arrives. However, watch for the vehicles arrival. It may be a van or a car with Blue Cab markings. The driver cannot wait more than two minutes for you.

If you decide not to take NightRide after you have requested a trip, please call 734-528-5432 and cancel the trip request.

What It Costs

$5.00 standard fare per trip, cash only.

Online local newspapers, newsletters and other local news sources

University Record http://record.umich.edu/
The Michigan Daily http://www.michigandaily.com/
Ann Arbor News http://www.mlive.com/ann-arbor/
The Detroit Free Press http://freep.com/
The Detroit News http://www.detnews.com/
WDIV Local 4 – NBC http://www.clickondetroit.com/
WJBK Channel 2 – FOX http://www.myfoxdetroit.com/
WXYZ Channel 7 – ABC http://www.wxyz.com/
WWJTV CBS News http://wwjtv.com/

Events and things to do

Ann Arbor Convention and Visitors Bureau - The official tourism
    site www.annarbor.org
Ann Arbor Observer www.arborweb.com
Current http://ecurrent.com/

Matthaei Botanical Gardens and Nichols Arboretum http://www.
lsa.umich.edu/mbg/
Arts & Culture http://arts.umich.edu/
The Ark (live music shows) http://www.theark.org/
Nightclubs http://annarborobserver.com/cg/t9168.html

Medical Center internal floor maps

http://www2.med.umich.edu/healthcenters/gmaps/internal/
index.cfm

International Center

http://internationalcenter.umich.edu/

Exercise and Fitness

Central Campus Recreation Building (closest to Hospital)
https://recsports.umich.edu/article/central-campus-recreation-
building-ccrb

North Campus Recreation Building (closest to ICC – closed until
Fall 2018)
https://recsports.umich.edu/article/north-campus-recreation-
building-ncrb

Outdoor Adventures
https://recsports.umich.edu/outdooradv

Swimming Facilities
https://recsports.umich.edu/buildingandpoolhours

Runner's Map
http://www.mapmyrun.com/us/ann-arbor-mi/

Canoeing
http://www.michigan.org/Things-to-Do/Paddle-Sports/Canoeing/
    Default.aspx?city=G2767

YMCA
https://www.annarborymca.org/join/

Worship Services

Temples and Synagogues
http://businessfinder.mlive.com/MI-Ann-Arbor/Temples-and-
    Synagogues

Christian Churches
http://businessfinder.mlive.com/MI-Ann-Arbor/Christian-Churches

Churches – Other
http://businessfinder.mlive.com/MI-Ann-Arbor/Churches-Other

Bicycle rental

http://campusstudentbikeshop.com/
https://recsports.umich.edu/bluebikes

Shopping

In Ann Arbor
Briarwood Mall http://www.simon.com/mall/briarwood-mall
Arborland Center http://www.amcap.com/properties/
    arborland.html
Kerrytown http://kerrytown.com/
Downtown Ann Arbor http://mainstreetannarbor.org/
Arbor Hills: http://shoparborhills.com/

<u>Second hand items:</u>

Kiwanis: http://www.kiwanissale.com
Goodwill: http://www.shopgoodwilldetroit.com
Salvation Army: http://www.http://centralusa.salvationarmy.org/
Ann Arbor PTO Thrift Shop: www.a2ptothriftshop.org
Ann Arbor Thrift Shop: www.annarborthriftshop.org
Treasure Mart www.treasuremart.com

Outlet malls outside of Ann Arbor

Tanger Outlets http://www.tangeroutlet.com/

Great Lakes Crossing Outlets http://www.greatlakescrossingoutlets. com/

Birch Run Premium Outlets http://www.premiumoutlets.com/ outlet/birch-run

Appendix 5

Faculty Email from Mark Schlissel 9 July 2017

Dear Colleagues:

We write today to address a serious and disturbing federal proposal that threatens the future of our work as the nation's most productive public research university. The proposal would reduce research funding by slashing reimbursements for facilities and administrative costs (F&A, also called indirect costs or overhead), forcing universities to cut jobs and shift research portfolios, jeopardizing our research mission.

Right now, this proposal is part of the administration's FY18 budget proposal and is also being considered by the White House and the U.S. Department of Health and Human Services for immediate implementation. Its scope includes grants awarded by the National Institutes of Health, which last year provided $457.3 million in support of faculty research at the University of Michigan. It could also be extended to other federal agencies that support university research. While there is strong bipartisan support for NIH funding in Congress, some members view a cap on F&A reimbursement as a politically palatable way to reduce federal expenditures on medical research.

We hope you can help us ensure that your colleagues and research partners fully understand the facts and consequences of this proposal, which are detailed further below. All NIH funded labs will feel the consequences of the proposed F&A cut.

Like you, we chose to work at a research university whose work advances the public good. The people who stand to lose most from the administration's proposal are our patients, our students, and the members of our community whose health is improved or whose lives are saved by the amazing research we do.

The F&A reimbursement proposal

When the NIH awards a grant to a university, the total cost includes two components:

- Direct costs fund expenses that can be attributed to individual projects. Examples include salary support for research staff and students, benefits, supplies, equipment, travel, and publication costs.
- F&A costs support crucial infrastructure, facilities and administrative investments and are essential for the conduct of the funded research. F&A costs cannot be assigned to a single project because they are items like laboratory space, heat, lights, IT infrastructure, library collections, grant accounting, purchasing, journal subscriptions (electronic and print), animal care facilities, hazardous waste disposal, security, insurance, and the support staff required to ensure compliance with a complex array of federal and state regulations.

The White House proposal would impose a 10 percent cap on F&A cost reimbursements to the university's NIH grants. Currently, F&A costs are established in partnership with the federal government using long-existing guidelines that ensure accountability of all parties. The proposed cap on NIH reimbursements would result in about $92 million in lost funding to U-M.

There is often a misconception that F&A costs do not directly support research. Characterizing F&A costs as "indirect" is imprecise. These vital funds are used to partially reimburse universities for investments that are essential to the support of quality research. The actual costs are much higher.

To fully consider the impact of the proposed cut, we describe how U-M's current F&A reimbursement rate – which is based on actual audited costs historically incurred by the university – is negotiated with the federal government, as well as explain some of the possible consequences for both our campus and the society we serve.

References

Articles

Abedini NC, Danso-Bamfo S, Moyer C, Danso KA, Makiharju H, Donkor P, Johnson TRB, Kolars JC. Perceptions of Ghanaian medical students completing a clinical elective at the University of Michigan Medical School. Acad Med. 89(7):1014–1017, 2014.

Abedini NC, Danso-Bamfo S, Kolars JC, Danso KA, Donkor P, Johnson TRB, Moyer CA. Cross-cultural perspectives on the patient-provider relationship: a qualitative study exploring reflections from Ghanaian medical students following a clinical rotation in the United States. BMC Medical Education. 15:161, 2015.

Adanu R, Obed S. Ruptured uterus at the Korle-Bu Teaching Hospital, Accra, Ghana. International journal of gynaecology and obstetrics: the official organ of the International Federation of Gynaecology and Obstetrics. 73: 253–255, 2001.

Adanu RMK. Cervical cancer knowledge and screening in Accra, Ghana. Journal of Women's Health & Gender-Based Medicine. 11:487–488, 2004.

Adanu RMK, Addington C, Cantor A, Johnson TRB. Publication ethics: Submissions to IJGO from low- and middle-income countries. Int J Gynecol Obstet. 38:1–2, 2017.

Altman, D, Carroli, G, Duley, L, Farrell, B, Moodley, J, Neilson, J, Smith, D, & Magpie Trial Collaboration Group. Do women with pre-eclampsia, and their babies, benefit from magnesium sulphate? The Magpie Trial: a randomised placebo-controlled trial. Lancet (London, England), 359(9321), 1877–90, 2002.

Amuakwa-Mensah F, Nelson AA. Retention of medical doctors in Ghana through local postgraduate training. J Educ Practice. 5:120–133, 2014.

Anderson FWJ, Mutchnick I, Kwawukume EY, Danso KA, Klufio CA, Clinton Y,Yun LL, Johnson TRB. Who will be there when women deliver? Assuring retention of obstetric providers. Obstet Gynecol. 110:1–5, 2007.

Anderson FWJ, Johnson TRBJ. U-M Medicine: Long-term Partnerships in Ghana. J Int Institute. 15(2):11, 2008.

Anderson FWJ, Wansom T. Beyond medical tourism: authentic engagement in global health. Virtual Mentor. 11(7):506–10, 2009.

Anderson F, Donkor P, de Vries R, Appiah-Denkyira E, Dakpallah GF, Rominski S, Hassinger J, Lou A, Kwansah J, Moyer C, Rana GK, Lawson A, Ayettey S. Creating a charter of collaboration for international university partnerships: the Elmina Declaration for Human Resources for Health. Academic medicine: journal of the Association of American Medical Colleges. 89(8):1125–1132, 2014.

Anderson FW, Obed SA, Boothman EL, Opare-Ado H. The public health impact of training physicians to become obstetricians and gynecologists in Ghana. Am J Public Health. 104(Suppl 1):S159–S165, 2014.

Anderson FWJ, Johnson TRB. Capacity building in obstetrics and gynaecology through academic partnerships to improve global women's health beyond 2015. BJOG. 122:170–173, 2014.

Anderson FWJ, Johnson TRB, DeVries R. Global Health Ethics: The Case of Maternal and Neonatal Survival. Best Practice & Research. Clinical Obstetrics and Gynecology. 43:125–135, 2017.

Andreatta P, Perosky J, Johnson TRB. Two-provider technique for bimanual uterine compression to control postpartum hemorrhage. J Midwifery Women's Health. 57(4):371–375, 2012.

Bediako-Bowan A, Yorke J, Brand N, Panzer K, Dally CK, Debrah S, Agbenorku P, Nkrumah Mills J, Huang LC, Laryea J, Lowry A, Appeadu-Mensah W, Adanu R, Kwakye G. Creating a Colorectal Surgery Fellowship in Ghana to Address the Growing Need for Colorectal Surgeons in West Africa. Dis Colon Rectum. 2023 Jun 23. doi: 10.1097/DCR.0000000000002996. Epub ahead of print.

Brewer TF, Saha N, Clair V. From boutique to basic: a call for standardised medical education in global health. Medical Education. 43:930–933, 2009.

Cherinet FM, Tekalign SY, Anbesse DH,Bizouneh ZY. Prevalence and associated factors of low vision and blindness among patients attending St. Paul's Hospital Millennium Medical College, Addis Ababa, Ethiopia. BMC Ophthalmol. 2018; 232(18).

Clinton HR, Obama B. Making patient safety the centerpiece of medical liability reform. N Engl J Med. 2006; 354:2205–2208.

Clinton Y, Anderson FW, Kwawukume EY. Factors related to retention of postgraduate trainees in obstetrics-gynecology at the Korle-Bu Teaching Hospital in Ghana. Acad Med. 85(10): 1564–1570, 2010.

Connors SC, Nyaude S, Challender A, Aagaard E, Velez C, Hakim J. Evaluating the Impact of the Medical Education Partnership Initiative at the University of Zimbabwe College of Health Sciences Using the Most Significant Change Technique. Acad Med. 2017 Sep; 92(9): 1264–1268.

Crump JA, Sugarman J. Ethical considerations for short-term experiences by trainees in global health. JAMA. 300(12):1456–1458, 2008.

Dalton VK, Xu X, Mullan P, Danso KA, Kwawukume Y, Gyan K, Johnson TRB. International family planning fellowship program: Advanced training in family planning to reduce unsafe abortion. Int Perspect Sex Reprod Health. 39(1):42–46, 2013.

Danso-Bamfo S, Abedini NC, Makiharju H, Danso KA, Johnson TRB, Kolars J, Moyer CA. Clinical electives at the University of Michigan from the perspective of Ghanaian medical students: A qualitative study. African Journal of Health Professions Education. 9(4):203–207, 2017.

Djulbegovic B, Guyatt GH. Progress in evidence-based medicine: a quarter century on. Lancet. 390(10092):415–423, 2017.

Dzomeku VM, van Wyk B, Lori JR. Experiences of women receiving childbirth care from public health facilities in Kumasi, Ghana. Midwifery. 55: 90–95, 2017.

Dzomeku, VM, Mensah, ABB, Nakua, EK, Agbadi P, Okyere J, Donkor P, Lori, JR. Promoting respectful maternity care: challenges and prospects from the perspectives of midwives at a tertiary health facility in Ghana. BMC Pregnancy Childbirth. 22: 451, 2022.

Erikson SL, Wendland C. Exclusionary practice: medical schools and global health clinical electives. BMJ. 348:g3252, 2014.

Erondu, NA, Aniebo, I., Kyobutungi, C., Midega J., Okiro E., Okunu F. Open letter to international funders of science and development in Africa. Nat Med. 27(5):742–744, 2021.

Essuman A, Gold KJ, Vitale C, Toma G, Cigolle C, Gyakobo M, Spangenberg K, Odoi-Gyarko K, Skye E, Zazove P. Establishing the First Geriatric Medicine Fellowship Program in Ghana: A Collaboration Between the University of Michigan and the Ghana College of Physicians and Surgeons. J Am Geriatr Soc. 67:1718–1723, 2019.

Fathalla MF. Human rights aspects of safe motherhood. Best Pract Res Clin Obstet Gynaecol. 20(3):409–419, 2006.

Heisel CJ, Fashe CM, Garza PS, Gessesse GW, Nelson CC, Tamrat L, Abuzaitoun R, Lawrence SD. Glaucoma Awareness and Knowledge Among Ethiopians in a Tertiary Eye Care Center. Ophthalmol Ther. 2021 Mar;10(1):39–50.

Heisel CJ, Garza PS, Fashe CM, Sime A, Nelson C. Normative Exophthalmometry Measurements Vary Among Ethiopian Adults and the Major Ethiopian Ethnic Groups. Ophthalmic Plastic and Reconstructive Surgery. 2020: 36:601-604.

Hessburg JP, Murthy P, Patel KD, Ostrowsk DP, Sienko KH. An assisted obstetric delivery device for resource limited settings. International Journal for Service Learning in Engineering. 7(2):1–12, 2012.

Hudspeth JC, Rabin TL, Dreifuss BA, Schaaf M, Lipnick MS, Russ CM, Autry AM, Pitt MB, Rowthorn V. Reconfiguring a One-Way Street: A Position Paper on Why and How to Improve Equity in Global Physician Training. Acad Med. 2019 Apr;94(4):482–489.

Jiagge E, Oppong JK, Bensenhaver J, Aitpillah F, Gyan K, Kyei I, Osei-Bonsu E, Adjei E, l Ohene-Yeboah M, Toy K, Jackson KE, Akpaloo M, Acheampong D, Antwi B, Agyeman FO, Alhassan Z, Fondjo LA, Owusu-Afriyie O, Brewer RN, Gyamfuah A, Salem B, Johnson T, Wicha M, Merajver S, Kleer C, Pang J, Amankwaa-Frempong E, Stark A, Abantanga F, Newman L, Awuah B. Breast cancer and African ancestry: Lessons learned at the ten-year anniversary of the Ghana-Michigan Research Partnership and International Breast Registry. J Glob Oncol. 2:302–310, 2016.

Johnson TRB. Implementing evidence-based science to improve women's health globally. Int J Gynecol Obstet. 122(2):91–93, 2013.

Kachalia A, Kaufman SR, Boothman R, Anderson S, Welch, K, Saint S, Rogers MAM. Liability Claims and Costs Before and After Implementation of a Medical Error Disclosure Program. Ann Intern Med. 153:213–221, 2010.

Kekulawala M, Johnson TRB. Ethical issues in global health engagement. Semin Fetal Neonatal Med. 23(1):59–63, 2018.

Kekulawala M, Samba A, Braunschweig Y, Plange-Rhule J, Turpin C, Johnson TRB, Anderson FWJ. Obstetric capacity strengthening in Ghana results in wide geographic distribution and retention of certified Obstetrician/ Gynaecologists: A quantitative analysis. BJOG: Int J Obstet Gy. 2022;129:1757–1761.

Klufio CA, Kwawukume EY, Danso KA, Sciarra JJ, Johnson T. Ghana postgraduate obstetrics/gynecology collaborative residency training program: Success story and model for Africa. Am J Obstet Gynecol. 189:692–696, 2003.

Kruk ME, Johnson JC, Gyakobo M, Agyei-Baffour P, Asabir K, Kotha SR, Kwansah J, Nakua, E, Snow RC, Dzodzomenyo M. Rural practice preferences among medical students in Ghana: A discrete choice experiment. Bull World Health Organ. 88(5):333–341, 2010.

Kuteesa J, Musiime V, Munabi I.G., Mubuuke AG, Opoka R, Mukunya D, Kiguli S. Specialty career preferences among final year medical students at Makerere University College of health sciences, Uganda: a mixed methods study. BMC Med Educ. 21:215, 2021.

Lane R. Profile: Senait Fisseha: empowering women through reproductive health. Lancet. 394(Oct 19):1405, 2019.

Lassey AT, Lassey PD, Boamah M. Career destinations of University of Ghana Medical School graduates of various year groups. Ghana Medical Journal. 47(2):87–91, 2013.

Lawrence ER, Moyer C, Ashton C, Ibine BAR, Abedini NC, Spraggins Y, Kolars J, Johnson TRB. Embedding international medical student electives within a 30-year partnership: the Ghana-Michigan collaboration. BMC medical education. 20(1):1–7, 2020.

Lawson JB. The Bight of Benin and beyond: reflections on obstetrics in the developing world. Int J Gynecol Obstet 34:101–105, 1991.

Lemmermen K, Van Wingen T, Scott P, Spencer C, Sienko KH. Adult male circumcision tool for use in traditional ceremonies. Journal of Medical Devices. 4(4):045003–0450037, 2010.

Lori JR, Rominski SD, Gyakobo M, Muriu EW, Kweku NE, Agyei-Baffour, P. Perceived barriers and motivating factors influencing student midwives' acceptance of rural postings in Ghana. Hum Resour Health. 10:17, 2012.

Luckett R, Nassali M, Melese T, Moreni-Ntshabele B, Moloi T, Hofneyr GJ, Chobanga K, Masunge J, Makhema J, Pollard M, Ricciotti H, Ramogola-Masire D, Bazzett-Matabele L. Development and launch of the first obstetrics and gynaecology master of medicine residency training programme in Botswana. BMC Medical Education. 21:19, 2021.

Mahler H. The Safe Motherhood Initiative: A Call to Action. Lancet. Mar 21:1(8534):668–670, 1987.

Maine D, Rosenfield A. The Safe Motherhood Initiative: Why has it stalled? Am J Pub Health. 89(4):480–482, 1999.

Martel J, Oteng R, Mould-Millman NK, Bell S, Zakariah A, Oduro G, Kowalenko T, Donkor P. The Development of Sustainable Emergency Care in Ghana: Physician, Nursing and Prehospital Care Training Initiatives. J Emerg Med. 47(4):462–468, 2014.

McLaren ZM, Sharp A, Hessburg JP, Sarvestani AS, Parker E, Akazili J, Johnson TRB, Sienko K. Cost effectiveness of medical devices to diagnose pre-eclampsia in low-resource settings. 2:99–106, 2017.

Mock CN, Donkor P, Gawande A, Jamison DT, Kruk ME, Debas HT; DCP3 Essential Surgery Author Group. Essential surgery: key messages from Disease Control Priorities, 3rd edition. Lancet, 2015: 385:2202–2219.

Mohedas I, Daly SR, Sienko KH. Design Ethnography in Capstone Design: Investigating Student Use and Perceptions. International Journal of Engineering Education. 30(4):888–900, 2014.

Mohedas I, Daly SR, Sienko KH. Requirements development: approaches and behaviors of novice designers. Journal of Mechanical Design. 2015; July;137(7).

Mohedas I, Kaufmann EE, Daly SR, Sienko KS. Ghanaian undergraduate biomedical engineering students' perceptions of their discipline and career opportunities. Global Journal of Engineering Education. 2015; 17(1):34–41.

Mohedas I, Sabet Sarvestani A, Bertch C, Franklin A, Joyce A, McCormick J, Shoemaker M, Bell C. Assistive Device for the Insertion of Subcutaneous Contraceptive Implants. Journal of Medical Devices. 2015; June;9(2).

Mould-Millman NK, Oteng R, Zakariah A, Osei-Ampofo M, Oduro G, Barsan W, Donkor P, Kowalenko T. Assessment of Emergency Medical Services in the Ashanti Region of Ghana. Ghana Med J. 2015; 49(3):125–135.

Natala N, Owusu-Antwi R, Donnir G, Kusi-Mensah K, Burns H, Mohiuddin S, Fluent T, Riba M, Dalack G. Building Child and Adolescent Psychiatry Expertise in Ghana Through Training and Knowledge Dissemination: a Review of the Initial Collaboration Stages, Opportunities, and Challenges. Curr Psychiatry Rep. 20:105, 2018.

Nordling L. (2017, March 17). San people of Africa draft code of ethics for researchers. Science.

Olatunbosun O. A practical guide to obstetrics in the tropics [Review of the book *Comprehensive Obstetrics in the Tropics,* by E.Y. Kwawukume & E. E. Emuveyan]. Lancet. 360(9337):956–957, 2002.

Osei-Ampofo M, Oduro G, Oteng R, Zakariah A, Jacquet G, Donkor P. The evolution and current state of emergency care in Ghana. African Journal of Emergency Medicine. 2013;3:52–58.

Osei-Ampofo M, Tafoya MT, Tafoya CA, Oteng R, Ali H, Becker TK. Skill and knowledge retention after training in cardiopulmonary ultrasound in Ghana: an impact assessment of bedside ultrasound training in a resource-limited setting. Emerg Med J. 2018;35:704–707.

Oteng R, Arhin B, Boakye-Yiadom J, Goldstick J, Eastman MR, Maio RF. A distance clinical research training course in Ghana. Int J Acad Med. 2020;6:209–14.

Oteng, R, Donkor P. The Ghana Emergency Medicine Collaborative. Academic Medicine. 2014;89(8):S110-S111.

Oteng RA, Osei-Kwame D, Forson-Adae MSE, Ekremet K, Yakubu H, Arhin B, Maio R. The preventability of trauma-related death at a tertiary hospital in Ghana: a multidisciplinary panel review approach. African Journal of Emergency Medicine. 2019;9:202–206.

Parikh SM. Global health ethics and professionalism education at medical schools. AMA J Ethics. 12(3):197–201, 2010.

Perosky JE, Rabban RN, Bradshaw JGT, Gienapp AP, Ofosu AA, Sienko KH. Designing a portable gynecological examination table: Improving access to antenatal care in rural Ghana. International Journal for Service Learning in Engineering. 7(1):1–14, 2012.

Peterson, HB; d'Arcangues C; Haidar, J; Curtis KM; Merialdi M; Gülmezoglu AM; Say L; Mbizvo M. Accelerating Science-Driven Solutions to Challenges in Global Reproductive Health: A New Framework for Moving Forward. Obstetrics & Gynecology. 117:720–726, 2011.

Peterson HB; Haidar J; Fixsen D; Ramaswamy R; Weiner BJ. PhD; Leatherman, S. Implementing Innovations in Global Women's, Children's, and Adolescents' Health: Realizing the Potential for Implementation Science. Obstetrics & Gynecology. 131:423–430, 2018.

Rominski SD, Lori J, Nakua E, Dzomeku V, Moyer CA. "When the baby remains there for a long time, it is going to die so you have to hit her small for the baby to come out": justification of disrespectful and abusive care during childbirth among midwifery students in Ghana, Health Policy and Planning. 32(2):215–224, 2017.

Rominski, SD, Yakubu, J, Oteng, RA, Peterson, M, Tagoe, N. Bell SA: The role of short-term volunteers in a global health capacity building effort: the Project HOPE-GEMC experience. Int J Emerg Med 8: 23, 2015.

Rosenfield A, Maine D. Maternal Mortality—a neglected tragedy: Where is the M in MCH? Lancet. Jul 13;2(8446):83–85, 1985.

Sabet Sarvestani A, Sienko KH. Design ethnography as an engineering tool. DEMAND: ASME Global Development Review. 1(2), 2014.

Sai FT, Measham DM. Safe Motherhood Initiative: Getting our priorities straight. Lancet. 339:478–480, 1992.

Shah S, Wu T. The medical student global health experience: professionalism and ethical implications. J Med Ethics. 34:375–378, 2008.

Sienko KH, Kaufmann EE, Musaazi M, Sabet Sarvestani A, Obed S. Obstetrics-based clinical immersion of a multinational team of biomedical engineering students in Ghana. International Journal of Obstetrics & Gynecology. 127:216-220, 2014.

Sienko KH, Sabet Sarvestani A, Grafman L. Medical device compendium for the developing world: a new approach in project and service-based learning for engineering graduate students. Global Journal of Engineering Education. 15(1), 2013.

Sienko KH, Young MR, Kaufmann EE, Obed S, Danso, KA, Opare-Addo HS, Odoi, AT, Turpin CA, Konney TO, Abebe Z, Mohedas I, Huang-Saad A, Johnson TRB. Global Health Design: Clinical Immersion, Opportunity Identification and Definition, and Design Experiences. International Journal of Engineering Education. 34(2(B)): 780–800, 2018.

Sokol D. Aequanimitas. BMJ. 335(7628):1049, 2007.

Stagg AR, Blanchard MH, Carson SA, Peterson HB, Flynn EB, Ogburn T. Obstetrics and Gynecology Resident Interest and Participation in Global Health. Obstet Gynecol. 129(5):911–917, 2017.

Starrs AM. Safe Motherhood Initiative: 20 years and counting. Lancet. 368:1130–1132, 2006.

Taylor CE. Ethics for an international health profession. Science. 153:716–720, 1966.

Tita AT, Stringer JSA, Goldenberg RL, Rouse DJ. Two decades of the Safe Motherhood Initiative: time for another wooden spoon award? Obstet Gynecol. 110(5):972–976, 2007.

Toma G, Essuman A, Fetters MD. Family medicine residency training in Ghana after 20 years: resident attitudes about their education. Fam Med Community Health. 2020. Oct;8(4):e000394.

Trimble EL, Helzlsouer KJ. Strengthening global partnership in breast cancer research. J Glob Oncol 2(5):253–254, 2016.

Waller B, Larsen-Reindorf R, Duah M, Opoku-Buabeng J, Edwards BM, Brown D, Moyer J, Prince M, Basura GJ, Otolaryngology outreach to Komfo Anokye Teaching Hospital: a medical and educational partnership. Journal of Laryngology & Otology. 31:608–613, 2017.

Winget CO, Fisher TK, Kumar RN, Harrington AH, Henke G, Davenport RD, Odoi AT, Sienko KH. Blood salvage device for use during ruptured ectopic pregnancy in low-resource countries. Int J Gynaecol Obstet. Jan;128(1):74–75, 2015.

Chapters in Books

Johnson CT, Johnson TRB. Ethical issues for global surgical engagement: the case of obstetric surgery. In: Jacobs LA: Practical ethics for the surgeon. Wolters Kluwer, Philadelphia 2018. Pages 161–165.

Johnson CT, Johnson T, Adanu RMK. Obstetric Surgery. In: Debas H, Gawande A, Jamison D, Kruk M (eds.): Disease Control Priorities, 3rd Edition, vol. 2 Essential Surgery, Chapter 5, 2015. Pages 77–94 Washington, DC: The International Bank for Reconstruction and Development / The World Bank.

Punch, J. How to Train Surgical Subspecialists in Sub-Saharan Africa. In: Hardy, M.A., Hochman, B.R. (eds): Global Surgery: How to Work and Teach in Low- and Middle-Income Countries. N.p.: Springer Cham, 2023. Pages 87–95.

Silverman RA. Locating culture with/in a Ghanaian Community. In: Silverman RA (ed.): Museum as Process: Translating local and Global Knowledges. London: Routledge, 2015. Pages 208–227.

Spector-Bagdady, Johnson TRB. Ethical Issues in Academic Global Reproductive Health. In: Chor J and Watson K (eds.): Reproductive Ethics in Clinical Practice: Preventing, Initiating, and Managing Pregnancy and Delivery—Essays Inspired by the MacLean Center for Clinical Medical Ethics Lecture Series. Oxford: Oxford University Press, 2021. Pages 247–261.

Books

Aellah G, Chantler T, Geissler PW. Global Health Research in an Unequal World: Ethics case studies from Africa. Oxfordshire, UK: CAB International, 2016.

Anderson FJ, ed. Building Academic Partnerships to Reduce Maternal Morbidity and Mortality: A Call to Action and Way Forward. Ann Arbor, MI: University of Michigan Press, 2014.

Anderson FWJ, ed. Eliminating Preventable Maternal and Neonatal Morbidity and Mortality: Critical Components in Building Capacity. Ann Arbor, MI: University of Michigan Press, 2016.

Biehl J, Petryna A, eds. When People Come First: Critical Studies in Global Health. Princeton, NJ: Princeton University Press, 2013.

Bossidy L, Charan R: Execution: The Discipline of Getting Things Done. New York: Random House, 2002.

Farmer P. Kim JY, Kleinman A, Basilico M, eds. Reimagining Global Health: An Introduction. Oakland: University of California Press, 2013.

Johnson CT, Hallock JL, Bienstock JL, Fox HE, Wallach, EE, eds. The Johns Hopkins Manual of Gynecology and Obstetrics. 5th ed. Baltimore: Lippincott Williams & Wilkins, 2015.

Kidder, T. Mountains Beyond Mountains: The Quest of Dr. Paul Farmer, a Man Who Would Cure the World. New York: Random House, 2003.

Klufio CA. An Introduction to Medical Statistics and Research. Accra: Woeli Publishing Services, 2003.

Kwawukume, EY, Emuveyan, EE. Comprehensive Obstetrics in the Tropics. Damsona: Ashante and Hittscher, 2002.

Kwawukume EY, Emuveyan EE. Comprehensive Gynaecology in the Tropics; Accra: Graphics Packaging, 2005.

Lasker, J. Hoping to Help: The Promises and Pitfalls of Global Health Volunteering. Ithaca: Cornell University Press, 2016.

Lawson JB, Harrison KA. Lawson & Stewart's Obstetrics and Gynaecology in Tropics and Developing Countries. 2nd ed. London: Hodder Arnold H&S, 1995.

Lawson JB, Harrison KA, Bergstrom S. Maternity Care in Developing Countries. London: RCOG Press, 2001.

Lawson JB, Stewart DB. Obstetrics and Gynaecology in the Tropics and Developing Countries. London: Edward Arnold Publishers, 1967.

Lucas AO. It Was the Best of Times…from local to global health. The Autobiography of Adetokunbo O. Lucas. Ibadan: BookBuilder Editions Africa, 2010.

National Academies of Sciences, Engineering and Medicine. Exploring Partnership Governance in Global Health: Proceedings of a Workshop. Washington DC: National Academies Press, 2018.

Nour N. Obstetrics and Gynecology in Low-Resource Settings: A Practical Guide. Boston: Harvard University Press, 2016.

Packard RM: A History of Global Health: Interventions into the Lives of Other Peoples. Baltimore: John Hopkins University Press, 2016.

Rosenfield PL. A World of Giving: Carnegie Corporation of New York— A Century of International Philanthropy. New York: New York: Public Affairs, 2014.

Silverman RA, Probst P, Abungu G. National Museums in Africa: Identity, History, and Politics. London: Routledge, 2021.

Wall AE. Ethics for International Medicine: A Practical Guide for Aid Workers in Developing Countries. Hanover NH: Dartmouth College Press, 2012.

Wendland CL. A Heart for the Work: Journeys through an African Medical School. Chicago: University of Chicago Press, 2010.

Websites

Asediba G. (2022, May 2). INSIGHTFUL DISCUSSION ON MORTUARIES (The horrible state of Korlebu Mortuary) [Video]. YouTube. https://www.youtube.com/watch?v=9hNt6veN2Zc

Emmanuel Quaye Archampong. (2023, April 21). In Wikipedia. https://en.wikipedia.org/wiki/Emmanuel_Quaye_Archampong

Michigan Medicine. (2016, November 22). Colonialism or Collaboration? https://www.michiganmedicine.org/medicine-michigan/colonialism-or-collaboration

Sujal Parikh. (2023, July 12). In Wikipedia. https://en.wikipedia.org/wiki/Sujal_Parikh

Undergraduate Research Opportunity Program. (2020, October 14). Yaera Spraggins, Recently Published UROP Alumni. https://lsa.umich.edu/urop/news-events/all-news/search-news/yaera-spraggins-urop-alumni-recently-published.html

Author Biography

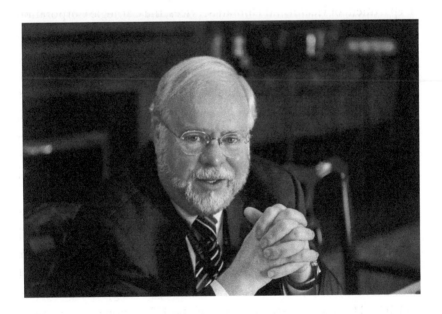

Timothy Robert Bradley Johnson received his education and training at the University of Michigan, University of Virginia, and Johns Hopkins University. After service in the US Air Force, he rejoined the Johns Hopkins faculty to eventually become director of the Division of Maternal-Fetal Medicine and chief of obstetrics. He served as Bates Professor of the Diseases of Women and Children and chair of the

Department of Obstetrics and Gynecology at the University of Michigan from 1993 to 2017 and continues there as Arthur F. Thurnau Professor of Obstetrics and Gynecology, Professor of Women's and Gender Studies, and faculty in the Center for Bioethics and Social Sciences in Medicine. For a time, he was interim director of Global REACH, the UM Medical School's international program, where he remains active. He is a fellow of the American College of Obstetricians and Gynecologists (ACOG) and fellow of the American Institute of Ultrasound in Medicine. While he was chair of the Department of Obstetrics and Gynecology at the University of Michigan, the department's national rankings in obstetrics and gynecology and women's health reached well into the "top ten" by the National Institutes of Health (NIH) and US News & World Report metrics. He received research and training grants from the NIH, the Department of Health and Human Services, the Carnegie Corporation of New York, and others. His research interests include fetal behavior, prenatal care, assessment and prevention of sexual harassment in academic medicine, medical education and capacity building for health, global women's health, and global health ethics. Doctor Johnson is active in international teaching and training, especially in Ghana, and he is an honorary fellow of the West African College of Surgeons, honorary fellow of the Ghana College of Surgeons, honorary fellow of the International College of Surgeons, and fellow ad eundem of the Royal College of Obstetricians and Gynaecologists (London). He has authored over three hundred articles, chapters, and books; he has served on numerous editorial boards, study sections, professional committees, and society and association boards; and he is past editor of the *International Journal of Gynecology and Obstetrics*, the official journal of the International Federation of Gynecology and Obstetrics (FIGO). He is an elected member of the US National Academy of Medicine. He has received the President's Award for Distinguished Service in International Education from the University of Michigan; the Distinguished Service Award, the highest honor of ACOG; the Distinguished Merit Award, the highest recognition of FIGO; and two honorary doctorates. He has received numerous honors for his teaching and is past president of the Association of Professors of Gynecology and Obstetrics. He has three children, six grandchildren, and lives with his wife in Ann Arbor, Michigan, where he continues to practice medicine, teach, and mentor, is active in community outreach and service, and enjoys the outstanding sports and arts offerings.